Daniela Danna

CONTRACT CHILDREN

Questioning Surrogacy

Daniela Danna

CONTRACT CHILDREN

Questioning Surrogacy

ibidem-Verlag
Stuttgart

Bibliografische Information der Deutschen Nationalbibliothek
Die Deutsche Nationalbibliothek verzeichnet diese Publikation in der Deutschen Nationalbibliografie; detaillierte bibliografische Daten sind im Internet über http://dnb.d-nb.de abrufbar.

Bibliographic information published by the Deutsche Nationalbibliothek
Die Deutsche Nationalbibliothek lists this publication in the Deutsche Nationalbibliografie; detailed bibliographic data are available in the Internet at http://dnb.d-nb.de.

Cover picture: Nosnibor137/bigstockphoto.com

∞

Gedruckt auf alterungsbeständigem, säurefreien Papier
Printed on acid-free paper

ISBN-13 Paperback edition: 978-3-8382-0760-5
ISBN-13 Hardcover edition: 978-3-8382-0810-7

© *ibidem*-Verlag
Stuttgart 2015

Alle Rechte vorbehalten

Das Werk einschließlich aller seiner Teile ist urheberrechtlich geschützt. Jede Verwertung außerhalb der engen Grenzen des Urheberrechtsgesetzes ist ohne Zustimmung des Verlages unzulässig und strafbar. Dies gilt insbesondere für Vervielfältigungen, Übersetzungen, Mikroverfilmungen und elektronische Speicherformen sowie die Einspeicherung und Verarbeitung in elektronischen Systemen.

All rights reserved. No part of this publication may be reproduced, stored in or introduced into a retrieval system, or transmitted, in any form, or by any means (electronic, mechanical, photocopying, recording or otherwise) without the prior written permission of the publisher. Any person who does any unauthorized act in relation to this publication may be liable to criminal prosecution and civil claims for damages.

Printed in Germany

Alla mia mamma

Contents

Introduction 9

CHAPTER 1) Familial constellations 19

What is surrogacy? 19

First BIG question: Who is the mother? 26

Actors in the agreement 32

Second BIG question: Whom does a newborn belong to? 41

Chapter 2) From conception to the baby 51

Fertilization and the beginning of pregnancy 51

The "pregnancy results" 56

Delivery and detachment 59

Chapter 3) Baby and the law 67

From status to contract 67

The contract versus the agreement 75

Regulations and slippery slopes 86

Suspended babies 99

Human rights of surrogacy babies 109

Chapter 4) Mothers and others 119
    The subjective experience 119
    Are they workers? 129
    Bad women 144
    Money making 149
    Relationships and conflicts 159

Conclusion: ethical surrogacy 173

References 185

Introduction

We women have long been struggling to maintain power over our capacity to give birth. In the *très longue durée* since the defeat of matriarchy (if it had ever existed), more and more of us across the planet have regained this power, becoming able to choose if and when to have children. Reproductive rights are the legal expression of this regaining our procreative capacities. The goal of reproductive rights for all women was stated in the Convention for the Elimination of All Forms of Discrimination against Women (CEDAW) adopted in 1979, and in all subsequent and related international treaties under the aegis of the UN. Reproductive rights, put into national laws and then into effect by an increasing number of countries, include the right for women "to decide freely and responsibly on the number and spacing of their children and to have access to the information, education and means to enable them to exercise these rights." In Beijing in 1995 it was made explicit that: "Acts of violence against women also include forced sterilization and forced abortion, coercive/forced use of contraceptives, female infanticide and prenatal sex selection" (Platform of Action for the Beijing Declaration).

How will women who have regained power over the birthing process decide to use it? If a woman uses it to have a child in order to help the infertile, will it mean that she has enslaved herself again with her own hands? Is it different whether she takes money for this act or not? What about the reimbursement of her expenses, what about her foregone gains? Should she be able to decide by herself on the destiny of a child born to her even if it was conceived by agreement? When should she decide his or her family destination? Moreover: what is the role of the concrete conditions of inequality in the present world-economy for the use that women make of their reproductive capacities? Generalizations are difficult: my point of view is from a core country, where women who cannot themselves bear children (or men) can utilize their other powers to ask a woman to bear a child for them—and not from a periphery or semiperiphery country where women are often asked to work in this way (countries of the "core" are richer as a result of their unequal exchange with the world's peripheries, in world-systems analysis terminology—see the works of Immanuel Wallerstein, Terence Hopkins, Giovanni Arrighi and their social science school).

I am writing this book to make a contribution to the debate, striving to preserve and enhance women's rights over our natural reproductive powers, within the context of all the new possibilities that reproductive technologies have brought about since the first successful birth of a baby conceived in vitro in 1978 (she was called Luise Brown). But technology is not involved in the minimal definition of the practice of surrogacy, which is basically the surrendering of a child after its birth to those who arranged for the pregnancy of the willing woman to take place. Or maybe, as in the Bible, who imposed the pregnancy on a slave. In fact, many authors point out that the—rather unfortunate—beginnings of surrogacy go as far back as the Old Testament. The Book of Genesis tells that Sarai, at 75, was too old to give the slightly younger Abram the progeny that would constitute Yahweh's people of the covenent. She suggested that Abram should make Hagar pregnant, and then she would raise the child as her own. Hagar was a slave in Abram's house, therefore not really entitled to express her opinion about the procedure. She gave a son to Abram, and Sarai became Ishmael's social mother, but only until she herself became pregnant and gave birth to their true heir Isaac. At that point, not only Abraham and Sarah got h's in their names, but both Hagar and Ishmael were thrown out of the house and sent into the wilderness, since her contribution to the construction of the new nation was no longer needed. In another passage from the Book of Genesis we can also find references to the direct purchase of children: "Every male among you who is eight days old must be circumcised, including those born in your household or bought with money from a foreigner," are Yahweh's reported words. Another biblical story of surrogacy involves two female slaves, Bilhah and Silpah, belonging to the sisters Rachel and Leah, with a partially unhappy ending: the second sister did not recognize the two sons that Silpah bore for her (Genesis 30).

In patrilinear societies, as legitimacy is conferred upon the child by the father, a male heir is strongly desired. Children were easily circulated from fertile to infertile couples in the extended family or beyond it. Now we have progress to help in procuring heirs with medical interventions, and infertility has become surmountable for many. Not having one's own children has become the difficult decision of when to stop medical interventions—however uncertain, costly, and painful they are.

Fostered by IVF technology (in vitro fertilization), surrogate agreements have seen a fast growth, similar to what happened when single heterosexual and lesbian women started having children *en masse* making recourse to assisted insemination with frozen sperm. There has always been the possibility to procreate with casual sex with a man, or with self-insemination, the low-tech, DIY option of inserting sperm into the vagina without sexual relations or medical intervention (a turkey baster does it). But only a minority conceives in these ways. Instead of community organizing to find donors and to secure anonymity (if wished for), and instead of going through the inconvenience of having casual sex with an untested stranger, paying doctors looks simpler and is therefore preferred—as it is by heterosexual couples, who could also practice self-insemination. We are used to delegating responsibility for our acts to "experts." But the reverse side is the application of more and more technology to the pregnancy and birthing process. As Caterina Botti conveys it: the main character at birth is not the woman becoming a mother, but the medical personnel—or rather the gynaecologist (Botti 2007). And in surrogate motherhood the main character it's not the pregnant woman at all, but the phantom of a child coming from nowhere, concretely manufactured by a clinic or by the services of an intermediating agency.

Women themselves perceive their bodies as fragile and inapt. On the contrary, no less than 80% of women (an estimate made by the gynecologists of IRIS, an Italian association promoting the rights to health and wellbeing) are able to give birth without complications—not really by themselves, but with the assistance of a midwife and of the pregnant woman's "birth team" of her choice.[1] But only a minority of women are confident enough in their natural powers to make this choice. The way in which women experience their pregnancy and delivery is increasingly a surrender to the experts' advice, a constant relationship with doctors instead of making recourse to medicine only if in need, and the acceptance of any technological intervention, useful or not. For instance, both in developed and developing

---

[1] See the works of Michel Odent, Frederick Lamaze, Clare Scropetto, Anni Daulter, Anita Regalia (among others). A midwife from Sardinien testifies about the easy pre-medicalization birthing process: "An obstetrician who started working as an assistant in the '60s remembers that she assisted about 360 deliveries in six years, of which two were hospitalized because of the fetal presentation. She had to perform episiotomy in just one case, rarely used spartina, and never ossitocin" (Centro studi 1985, 4; my translation, as for all the other quoted texts not originally in English). Episotomy and lacerations were avoided by massage with oil and by the midwife sustaining the perineum with her hand.

countries, women increasingly lie in bed in the gynecological position at delivery (Makuch 2010). This position is comfortable only for the clinicians who supervise the delivery (in fact gynecologists invented it, putting the gestatorial chair away in the attic).[2] But it is doubtful that women would choose it, as it contrasts gravity and makes the descent of the fetus through the birth canal much more difficult than any other position—except being hung upside down.

Are the technological novelties enhancing women's freedom, solving the infertility problems of those who do not possess procreative natural power, or are they just a deceptive device to deprive women of what used to be a unique experience and a unique tie between mother and child? We stand at a crossroad.

The preamble of the Convention for the Elimination of All Forms of Discrimination against Women stresses "that a change in the traditional role of men as well as the role of women in society and in the family is needed to achieve full equality of men and women." New reproductive techniques, in particular IVF plus implant of the fecundated egg, certainly amount to an abrupt change in traditional gender roles: the fragmentation of the "mother" is the most commented upon of its features. Since 1978 we must distinguish between egg, pregnancy, and social motherhood on one hand, and on the other (as also in former times) between sperm and social fatherhood. The Convention on the Rights of the Child (1989) recognizes the child's right to grow up with her or his family, and also the European Convention for Human Rights has codified a right to the respect of one's "family life," but the new technologies have confused the scene, and many now have doubts about what the family of a child conceived in vitro with a donor egg really is. Among genes, intentions and pregnancy, what and who decides?

I will show how the doubts about what the child's family is and who her or his mother is rather derive from a linguistic sleight of hand, because "mother" is not the feminine for "father," and vice versa. The doubts can grow on this (literal) "gender" confusion, while the fundamental question is quite simple, looking at the existing relationships.

---

[2] At the IRIS Association Conference "Volti e risvolti della paura" (Milan 12.12.2014) the tale of a midwife was reported: "The gynecologist peered in and saw the woman in labor on all fours: 'Put her back in bed in a civilized position!' he told me" (in the original: "in una posizione da cristiani," an Italian set phrase).

Should we welcome the new techniques for this "gender deconstructive" effect? Can they work towards gender equality and against gender discrimination? Will it do good that a woman can freely give, or contract out her "gift of life" to others? Should not women be able to enter rational contracts, even if they entail the decision of conferring the child they bore to another family? Will the new possibilities help to stop the consideration of women as inferior to men, of men as superior to women?

Some commentators (Carmel Shalev, Marcela Iacub) welcome the deliberate detachment of pregnancy and motherhood, because they praise *contract* as a practice of the right to choose, even a marker for a democratic society, in opposition to *status*, representing all the oppressive ways of traditional society and the expression of the inescapable obligations imposed by "the power" over the individual. Others (Carole Pateman, Margaret Radin, Elizabeth Anderson) consider such a contract demeaning for women and entailing a sale of children, whose psychological foundations are damaged by having been bought. Others still (Gena Corea, Maria Mies, Janice Raymond, Phyllis Chesler) do not only protest the contract, but the agreement itself, showing how surrogacy exploits women and fosters false consciousness over its sacrifices, embraced as self-enhancing acts of giving. But I find it impossible to condemn all acts of surrogacy. It can be welcomed under certain conditions: to be voluntary and gratuitous, thus avoiding the slippery slopes that transform it into a (demeaning) job. I am simply advocating for the centrality of the pregnant woman, that is the mother, in the process of creation of families (see also Zipper and Sevenhuijsen 1987, Field 1988, Shanley 1993 and of course the works of Barbara Katz Rothman).

Families created through surrogate motherhood are growing exponentially. "Surrogate babies" are now a 5-digit figure, as the very beginnings of surrogacy are quite long ago. The lawyer Noel Keane invented the term in 1976 to broker the agreements. In 1984 the first surrogate motherhood agreement with an embryo transfer took place: the egg came from a woman without a uterus and was implanted in one of her friends (Utian et al. 1985). In the US, Gena Corea (1985) estimated that in the decade beginning from 1976, births by agreement were 75–100, and in a similar period of time (1977–1988) about 40 "surrogacy babies" came into the world in Australia, while in the UK the Brazier report (1988) estimated that 50–80 new babies were born every year out of 100–180 agreements. The estimates for Canada were of 118 babies born up to 1992. Up to that year the worldwide total could be 4,000 (Spitz 1996, 70).

In the U.S, the American Society for Reproductive Medicine estimates that 530 "surrogacy babies" were born in 2004 and 1,179 in 2011. McDermott (2012) estimates a lower number of about 750 births per year. India soon followed the US: in fact the second place where an IVF baby was born was Kolkata, also in 1978, just two months after Louise Brown (but the case is controversial, see Smerdon 2008, 19–20). Three thousand births were estimated to have taken place in India in the decade since 1994. In 2004 in the small city of Anand the now famous clinic of doctor Nayna Patel opened: it has facilities for half a hundred pregnant women. Until recently, 100–300 births were estimated to occur every year in India, half of them destined to the "export market," mainly the "Anglo-Saxon" countries: US, Australia, UK, Canada—especially to Indian families residing there (Smerdon 2008, 22). Now it is estimated that in the 350 Indian clinics which mainly specialize in surrogate motherhood, around 3,000 births occur every year, dwarfing all the EU countries. In the UK from 1995 to 2007 the transfers of parental authority recorded by authorities were between 33 and 50, then the number started rising, up to 149 in 2011, approximately a fifth of them to same sex couples—a possibility that became legal in 2010 (Crawshaw, Blyth and van Akker 2013). In France it is estimated that 100–200 "surrogate babies" are fetched from abroad every year (Perreau-Saussine and Sauvage 2013, 119), in the Czech Republic about 15 a year (Pauknerová 2013,108).

In Israel from 1996 to 2001 there were 108 applications for surrogacy made to its Approval Committee which accepted 90 of them, with 30 babies born in 22 deliveries. In the period 2001–2006 the applications were 360, with 287 approvals, and 156 babies in 125 deliveries: "By the end of 2010, the Committee had received a total of 723 applications, out of which 327 babies were born in 260 births" (Shakargy 2013, 243). In Russia surrogacy programs made a total of 430 IVF cycles in 2009, but this is just the number of embryo transfers effected, not of resulting pregnancies (Kahzova 2013, 312). A truly astonishing estimate comes from China, where—prohibition of surrogacy notwithstanding—there are estimated to have been 25,000 births from these agreements up to 2009, according to the *Southern Metropolis Weekly*—maybe just a journalist's exaggeration (Huo 2013, 93). But, numbers apart, the picture is quite different from that of a prohibitionist country:

> Though the Ministry of Public Health of the PRC banned surrogacy in 2001, underground surrogacy businesses are thriving in the world's most populous country. Today, there are numerous surrogacy agencies in mainland China, most of which are located in big cities such as Beijing, Shanghai, Guangzhou, Wuhan and so on. Notwithstanding the tight control over the Internet by the Chinese Government, the websites of such agencies can easily be accessed. In the city of Beijing where the author lives, surrogacy advertisements are posted along the streets. The Chinese Government seems to turn a blind eye to the underground surrogacy industry in spite of the prohibition of surrogacy arrangements. (Huo 2013, 97)

The debate about ethics and policies for surrogacy has raged for three decades now, since the famous legal case of Baby M, born in 1986 and disputed between the birth mother and the commissioning couple. Conflicts have arisen not only about the delivery of babies, but also about abortion/embryo reduction, control of the pregnant woman's lifestyle, unwanted babies because of the end of the intended parent's relationships or because the baby was handicapped. Judiciary disputes in transnational surrogacy can arise if the home country's laws have been broken by performing surrogacy abroad in permissive or corrupt countries, obtaining a birth certificate for the child that is invalid in the parents' country.

The fears expressed by feminists such as Gena Corea in *The Mother Machine* (1985), Maria Mies and Vandana Shiva in *Ecofeminism* (1993), and Barbara Ehrenreich in *The Worst Years of Our Lives: Irreverent Notes from a Decade of Greed* (1990) that the "work" of pregnancy would be outsourced to poor women in Third World countries, have now come true: Indian clinics have mastered embryo-transfer technology, and it is cheaper for infertile couples to go there and use a "baby farm" than bother with arrangements or contracts at home.[3] Corea also foresaw that rich women would prefer not to go through pregnancy themselves—while Margaret Atwood in her dystopian novel *A Handmaiden's Tale*, 1984, shows a near future where a despised class of breeders is assigned to reproduction. This is not (yet?) true, but the growing engagement of women in labor markets where maternity is discouraged contributes to the postponing of childbearing which becomes increasingly difficult with age.[4]

---

[3] Thanks to the Indian state that from 1992 has been incentivizing medical tourism by subsidies to high-tech clinics, while the majority of the population cannot access health care.

[4] Also Silvia Federici wrote in 1999: "We have also seen the development of baby farms, in which children are produced specifically for export, and the increasing employment of 'third world women' as surrogate mothers. Surrogacy, like adoption, allows women from the 'advanced' capitalist countries to avoid interrupting their career or jeopardizing their

But it is difficult to renounce having a child. Motherhood is still a battlefield to define femininity, a dangerous zone where various social meanings and social and economic interests are fighting. It is a territory only partially liberated. In the '70s Adrienne Rich denounced the patriarchal institution of motherhood, but kept its oppressive imperatives distinct from a woman's possibility to live this experience in a satisfying and creative way if she rebelled against the rules of this social institution. Only by refusing to live in its cage and in the cage of the nuclear family, by not accepting to be an object of medical interference and control, by being insubmissive to the rules of male-ruled society (patriarchal power, as Rich wrote) can a woman live the joys of pregnancy and motherhood in full: by freeing herself, she frees her children, too. The price to pay is to be considered "mother outlaws," as Andrea O'Reilly proudly baptized her web site dedicated to activism and study about motherhood, with the aim of restoring its naturally empowering function for women, and of combating the emotional blackmailing and guilt feelings arising when a woman does not sacrifice everything to her family: "Mother Outlaws recognize that mothers and children benefit when the mother lives her life, and practices mothering, from a position of agency, authority, authenticity and autonomy."[5]

Surrogacy is one of the arenas where social meanings of motherhood are defined. The situation of a "carrier mother" cannot be univocally described, as laws are different, attitudes towards the phenomenon vary, and debates are inflamed. Where are we now? How to define what happens in surrogacy situations both from the point of view of public policies and individual ethics? What if the actors do not agree on these definitions? Whose definition should prevail?

Let us start by charting the ground: What are the social and biological interactions that configure surrogate motherhood? This is the theme of the first chapter. How is surrogacy performed? How is it similar or different to other kinds of motherhood? The second chapter illustrates the answers to these questions. Then: what are the legal boundaries that permit or prohibit

---

health to have a child. In turn, 'Third World' governments benefit from the fact that the sale of each child brings foreign currency to their coffers; and the World Bank and the International Monetary Fund tacitly approve of this practice, because the sale of children serves to correct 'demographic excesses' and is in harmony with the principle that debtor nations must export all their resources from forests to human beings" (Federici 2012, 72).

[5] Quoted from the homepage of www.motheroutlaws.org accessed 14.11. 2014.

the practice? The third chapter explores laws and rules in a global overview. Finally, who are the participants in these social or economic exchanges, in particular the surrogate mothers? The fourth chapter answers this question. Is there a way of allowing surrogacy that respects the prerogatives and rights of all parties involved? The conclusion answers this final question, suggesting a public policy to deal with the matter.

My sources for this book are mainly textual: the vast existing literature (legal material and ethnographic accounts, plus the debates about ethics and politics) and a few formal interviews that I conducted in a very difficult field.

I warmly thank my few interviewees for the sharing of their experiences and ideas; Angela Greco, Laila Sage, Veruska Sabucco, Olivia Garavaglia, Marta Fontana for their assistance in the research; the exponents of the network in-Fercit, led by Venetia Kantsa, and of the COST action BIRTH for correspondence and info; the staff at the University of Milan library for their valuable information and help; Mary Ellen Lanczak for her correction of my not native English language, and finally my editor at **ibidem**, Jakob Horstmann, for his conviction about the feasibility of this book.

CHAPTER 1)
Familial constellations

What is surrogacy?

"Surrogate motherhood," or surrogacy, "gestation for others" in French, "motherhood by legal substitution" or "by proxy" in Italian, "gestation by legal substitution" in Spanish "motherhood by interposed person" in Greek, "innkeeper mother" in Hebrew, "borrow-motherhood" in German, "carry-motherhood" in Dutch,[6] is just one of the many ways for infertile couples or individuals to try to have a child, involving the help of a willing woman. Surrogate motherhood does not take place in only one way, but is a varied practice basically consisting in an agreement between different subjects (singles or couples of the same or the opposite sex) and a woman who bears a child for them. According to the agreement, the natural mother will then sever her parental ties to the newborn (at birth or soon thereafter) in favor of the intended parent(s), who then become the primary caretaker(s) of the child and also—by various procedures—its legal parent(s).

It is sought especially in cases of infertility of the woman if she has viable eggs. Generally the "surrogate mother" gets pregnant using the intended father's semen—but in surrogacy the intended parent(s) are not necessarily the genetic parent(s), nor must the intended mother necessarily be infertile or with health issues impeding her pregnancy. It is also the only way to obtain a child for gay men who do not want to share parenthood with a woman. Surrogacy is sometimes called "contractual pregnancy"—which is inappropriate because a valid contract is only a special case in surrogacy, as only few jurisdictions grant its validity to regulate the practice. In fewer still does it provide for the enforcement of the relinquishment of parental rights by the birth mother. As surrogacy can take place both with an (informal) understanding or with a (legal) contract, we will generally call it an agreement. The woman who bears a child for others can have various motives, as the specifications "commercial" vs "altruistic" surrogacy indicate.

---

[6] Respectively: gestation pour autrui, maternità di sostituzione or maternità per procura, gestación subrogada, παρένθετη μητρότητα, אם פונדקאית (em pundekait), Leihmutterschaft, draagmoederschap.

In the past, arrangements like these were unusual, since informal adoption was much easier and the "adulterous," out-of-wedlock pregnancies that constitute surrogacy agreements today were heavily stigmatized. In modern societies with rule of law, this arrangement can legally work only in three situations: if the surrogate mother is unmarried, otherwise her husband will automatically be registered as the father of the infant (though his paternity can be contested by the genetic father); if she can give birth anonymously; or if the law explicitly allows for the recognition of surrogacy arrangements. This means that surrogacy is possible not only in the absence of a norm regulating it, but even in situations of prohibition. The simplest way is when the birth mother does not recognize the child (if legally possible), allowing for its recognition by the genetic father, or when she figures as the legal mother, but *de facto* relinquishes the child to be reared by the genetic father and his spouse or partner. The Napoleon Code of 1805 allowed for "accouchement sous X" (delivery under anonymity), a possibility that has since been legal in France, Italy and Luxembourg, and recently introduced in Mexico, Germany, Austria, and the Netherlands.[7] "Safe haven" laws permit anonymous parturition in nearly all the US and in the Czech Republic. Under these provisions if the natural father—as the genetic father is commonly called—recognizes the child, his wife can become its legal mother. These countries are rather the exceptions. In countries based on common law, with a Birth Register, only the woman who gives birth can be the legal mother; and another woman can become a mother only by adoption, even if she is the wife of the natural father, and even—in contemporary times—if she is a genetic mother, that is, the egg contributor.

A very rare extra-judicial testimony of an early case of surrogacy comes from the '70s in the Netherlands.[8] Juliette Zipper and Selma Sevenhuijsen recount that a woman of the feminist movement gave birth to a child conceived with her single ex boyfriend on his behalf. The man then raised the child without a close mother figure. It was all perfectly legal, as he had the

---

[7] In France the number of "accouchements sous X" has risen, from 588 in 2005 to about 700 in 2010. The birth mother can step back from her decision for a period of two months (Villeneuve-Gokalp 2011).

[8] It is often claimed that surrogacy agreements are ancient and that they have always been practiced in a common way, but I did not find traces other than (or before) this mention, plus the stories reported by Noel Keane (see further). The famous Biblical episodes were not agreements but slave exploitation.

written permission of the mother to recognize the child, which in the Netherlands is requested when parents are not married. He later obtained sole custody. "We never considered her arrangement concerning parenthood a relevant issue for feminism," conclude the authors, who personally knew the people involved (Zipper and Sevenhuijsen 1987, 118).

This kind of surrogacy, which did not even have a name and now is called "traditional" surrogacy, had the beauty of simplicity: no splitting of the mother figure was yet possible. The woman carrying the child was universally recognized as its mother: half the genetic material was hers, she bore and gave birth. That she should renounce her prerogatives as a mother could not be taken for granted by the intended parent(s): the last word was hers. Where surrogacy is unrecognized or forbidden by law it is still like that: the agreements cannot be prohibited by contrary authorities since they go undetected.

It was the Michigan lawyer Noel Keane who invented the expression "surrogate motherhood" and popularized the practice in the US by setting up an agency for intermediation. He got the idea in 1976 from a piece of news regarding a gay man who had a child in San Francisco by a woman whom he paid 7,000 USD to be let alone in raising their offspring. Keane started in the same year: while the surrogates were reimbursed with 10,000 USD, his center got 7,500 USD just for intermediation and legal paperwork. He advertised it on the Phil Donahue television show and, even after the exposure of the dangers of these agreements in the Baby M case, which he had arranged, he found scores of willing "surrogates," whom he matched with infertile couples in intermediation centers all over the US.[9]

In the second half of the '70s, IVF and embryo transfer were engineered, and from the end of the '80s surrogacy increasingly involved the use of these assisted reproductive technologies (ART from now on). But to define surrogacy as just one ART among the others is completely mistaken, though indeed very common. One example is Ciccarelli and Beckham (2005, 49) calling it a "new technology." Sometimes surrogacy is even called a "treatment" for "infertility," which in fact is not an illness, since the infertile

---

[9] He also wrote a book about surrogacy: Keane, Noel and Dennis Breo Keane, *The Surrogate Mother*. Everest Publishers, 1981. In Keane's obituary in the New York Times, his son declared that he arranged the birth of 600 children, some of them named after him by the grateful parents (http://www.nytimes.com/1997/01/28/nyregion/noel-keane-58-lawyer-in-surrogate-mother-cases-is-dead.html).

body is *per se* absolutely healthy. Like most remedies for infertility, surrogacy is definitively not a therapy. A possible source of this confusion is that surrogacy agreements have been forbidden by the laws regulating ART in many countries, such as Italy, France, and Germany.

In sum, surrogacy is the arrangement to use a woman's bearing capacity, and essentially is neither an ART or a contract. Some authors already take for granted its use only to avoid pregnancy. This does not currently seem to be the norm, but could become a more frequent development.

Together with the use of donated gametes, surrogacy is called "third-party reproduction," a terminology that indicates that to overcome their couple infertility, the would-be parents need a third party, somebody who is biologically contributing without becoming a social parent. Still, "third-party reproduction" is a very questionable term, as it lumps together sperm donation, egg donation and surrogate motherhood. The procedures are of course very different: if the third party is a man, his contribution is his sperm, pleasurably detachable from the male body.[10] If the genetic third party is a woman, her egg must be accessed with laparoscopy under anesthesia. In surrogacy, despite the wide use of the disparaging synonym of "wombs for rent," a whole woman is needed to complete the pregnancy process, which is long, inconvenient, cumbersome, risky and painful at delivery and often also before it.[11]

In general, our much relished principle of equality between the sexes has no meaning in human reproduction. Not only is it inappropriate to use concepts of equality or equivalence between the sexes in their biological role in this matter, but, as our culture is so strongly pervaded by ideas and ideals of equality, we risk blinding ourselves to the evident lack of proportion in the male and female contribution to reproduction,. My discussion with a friend about surrogacy ended nonsensically when, answering my rather commonplace remark that men cannot have—in the meaning of "make"—children, so they should respect the will of women in this matter, she re-

---

[10] This often does not happen without shame because of the taboos surrounding masturbation. Rene Almeling (2011, 99 ff.) recounts other difficulties, such as the bodily discipline required by sperm donation in the US, to which donors must commit at least once a week. They also relate feelings of objectification.

[11] Twenty per cent of the women in a sample considered birthing pain as unbearable, 30% as severe, 35% moderate and 15% light (research quoted by Goberna 2013, 82. Original: Bonica, J. J. and J. S. McDonald "The pain of childbirth," in J. J. Bonica, *The management of pain*, 1990^2, Lea & Febiger, Philadelphia, pp. 1313-1343.

plied: "But that is not fair!" Her view implied that there is a right for men to procreate with their sperm: but who will have to fulfil the corresponding duty and how? The jurist John A. Robertson (1983a, 1983b, 1986[12]), an advocate of surrogacy contracts, argued that the US should apply the "equal protection" principle, inscribed in the Fourteenth Amendment to the Constitution, to surrogacy as it otherwise would discriminate among fertile and infertile individuals, and among these between infertile men and infertile women. He would like to configure a right to noncoital reproduction that would in parallell allow the artificial insemination of women to remedy men's infertility, and surrogate motherhood to remedy women's infertility.[13] Again, whose duty will it be to fulfil this hypothetical right? No one can be forced to contribute, either genetically or much less with their whole bodies (that is, with a woman's body) in order for somebody else to be able to become a parent. Not only is it impossible for such a right to exist (though, indeed, a right to reproduce through women's bodies has been asserted through most of history with the collective exploitation of women by men), but it would not even be advisable to introduce it in the present context of a growing human population, already consuming—in the most unequal way in all human history—half of the world's biomass resulting from photosynthesis (Pimentel 2001). This ecologically unsustainable situation should not be fostered with such a "right to reproduce" for those who are unable to do it without ART. The choice to be childfree should be celebrated as ecologically sound, relieving the infertile from their feelings of guilt, inadequacy and social failure—though of course the real remedy to the ecological crisis is to stop and change society's goal of capital accumulation, interrupting the capitalist D-M-D' circuit in favor of degrowth (e.g. Badiale and Bontempelli 2010).

The jurist Martha Fineman has dedicated her work as legal theorist to uncovering the problems that the diffuse legal culture of applying the equality principle between the sexes to family law have created:

---

[12] See also the detailed discussion of his arguments by Herbert Krimmel (1983, 12 ff.).
[13] The equality discourse pervades many "homoparenting" associations. They request: sperm donations for lesbians who want to become mothers and surrogate mothers for gay men who want to become fathers. It is a weak argument, and if challenged the answer is to back it up with sexist verbal violence (Famiglie Arcobaleno mailing list, 2007, on file with author).

> The evolution of de-gendered legal rules regulating families is more than a mere change in language reflecting the aspiration that all parents, male as well as female, will nurture and care for their children. Gender neutrality has substantive implications and signals a change in orientation in which caretaking is devalued and biological and economic connections are deemed of paramount importance. (Fineman 1995, 70)

She writes against "the gender-neutral fetish of liberal legalism," that does injustice to the mother/child relations in situations of divorce or forced recognition of fatherhood. She baptizes the current situation "the neutered mother." The influential idea of the interchangeability of parents has also symbolically had the pernicious consequence of canceling from our culture the recognition of female powers in reproduction, and the pregnant woman's unique relationship with the new life that she generated:

> an important component of the neutering process has been the designation of untraditional forms of motherhood as "pathological" or deviant. This stigmatizing process makes mothering outside of the context of a two-parent, traditional family susceptible to extensive legal regulation and supervision. Mother and child alone are incomplete and insufficient—the cause and perpetuators of social decay and decline. (Fineman 1995, 68, see also Fineman 2009)

A solution to these problems, according to Fineman, calls for a restructuring of our worldview because if we proceed from the idea that the cornerstone of society is an autonomous individual, we consider relations of dependency as exceptions, while they are the norm. We can find them not only in procreation but in illness, disability, old age. The whole process of social reproduction demonstrates the preeminence of dependency and care in the human relations that constitute society. Moreover, the history of late capitalism has proved that social justice is impossible to attain on the basis of the fiction of the "autonomous individual."

Similarly, taking a closer look at our idea of the family, we find that the two spouses occupy center stage: an adult man and an adult woman, both generally active in the labor market, plus only eventually their dependent children. Fineman calls this family concept "the sexual family," noting that its same-sex variant is increasingly getting legal and social recognition. But this definition of family extols autonomy and the sexual bond, excluding from its concept the necessary care to be given to dependents. The importance of care would be recognized if we adopted a different central image of the family, as basically composed of Mother and Child, a symbolic dyad exemplifying the basic ties of human dependency and care. This dyad should become our central idea of human interaction—what we call the family—while we should stop celebrating the individual (as he or she is autonomous only for a part of his or her life, and always vulnerable) and his or her voluntary sexual acts, which should not be of interest to the legislator. Fineman urges that the sexual bond must remain a private and free feature of social life, without foundational power in family law. How to organize one's sexual life should not be a concern of the state, and marriage—valuable as a private ceremony for those who believe in it—should not entail any legal value nor prescription. Besides, we must also note that not only the autonomous individual, but the sexual bond as well have proven fleeting, ephemeral, unpredictable—especially in contemporary circumstances, as the high and growing divorce rates demonstrate. The dependency bond generally lasts much longer and it is based on unforfeitable needs.[14]

The Mother/Child dyad is just a symbol (therefore the capital letters), standing for all situations of dependency and caregiving that constitute a family, and does not deny that men can be caretakers, too—though, regretfully, we do not see much of it in contemporary society. This dyad has also the cultural advantage of being an ancient symbol, and a contemporary reality, as more and more babies are born outside marriage bonds, raised by single mothers, while ex wives continue to be the main carer for the kids after a divorce.

The public support that in the US, where Fineman lives (but also elsewhere), is currently offered to couples, both materially and symbolically, should be better directed towards this true nucleus of human society. Single mothers are instead blamed for the ruin of America, while the sexual family is supported, for example, with tax reductions for the purchase of a home, splitting income for taxes, and all the similar benefits reserved to couples, that nobody questions or perceives as privileges—a fact analyzed and denounced also by the economist Nancy Folbre (2009). Exposure of the devaluation of care work in society and in social theory is a common theme for these authors and for the political campaigns started in the '70s by the feminist group Wages for Housework (see the works of Mariarosa Dalla Costa, Selma James, Silvia Federici). They theorize the profitability to capital not

---

[14] The dependency tie is indeed resented in the "sexual family." Hostility by the father to the mother/child relationship often occurs even in couples who had a good relationship before the arrival of a baby.

only of wage work, but of unwaged work, mainly performed by women in the family.

In implicit agreement with this political school of thought, Fineman is adamant that to substitute the current idea of the basic familial tie as a sexual tie between a woman and a man, with the dependency tie between Mother and Child should not mean that the social reproduction burden must always fall on mothers' shoulders (though there is a danger of this restrictive cultural interpretation). Responsibility to raise the next generation of human beings should be collectively assumed, helping the family (that is, basically the dyads) with public and collective services and benefits.

I can add that this revolutionary centering of the family on the Mother/Child relationship would have very important consequences on the way we both theorize and concretely deal with human ties, steering us in the direction of a renaissance of matrilinearity and matriarchy, as defined by Heide Göttner-Abendroth (e.g. 1980). Her studies on past and contemporary societies with matriarchal patterns describe egalitarian groups where women enjoy freedom—and not societies where power relations between the sexes are just reversed, as the name "matriarchy" would suggest if interpreted as simply the feminine form of "patriarchy." Were these ideas central to contemporary society, they would help to dispel our doubts about how to consider surrogacy—especially after the introduction of ART. Unfortunately we must start from the current and very different idea of the family as based on the sexual tie, so its concepts and labels must be deconstructed in order to be able to grasp what is really happening in surrogacy where ART are involved.[15]

First BIG question: Who is the mother?

As Karl Marx said, technology introduces new possibilities that re-arrange human existence and human relations. When reproductive technology enabled the implanting of embryos in wombs, even from another woman's ovum, the language of kinship acquired a new meaning, and the legal constructions based on it were called into question. The figure of the "mother,"

---

[15] Reality is a discredited word in contemporary social science, but we do not need an absolute concept. What is enough is a pragmatic and "incremental" concept, that is, the process of knowing has the aim of getting us closer to grasping reality, without the pretention of describing the truth once and for all.

already divisible into a birth-biological-genetic mother and a social one in the cases of formal or informal adoption and of "traditional" surrogacy, endured a further split. From then on, the birth mother, carrier of the embryo/fetus, could be a different woman from the one furnishing the genetic material, that is the egg. It appeared logical that the woman whose egg has been fertilized[16] should also be considered a "mother," entitled to share the attribution of biological motherhood with the birth mother who has carried the fetus to term. For example, the jurist Alicia Benedetta Faraoni (2002, 332–3) jokingly comments upon the "scientific revolution" that has called motherhood into question, saying that the famous Italian motto "di mamma ce n'è una sola" (the mother is only one—we have just one source of unconditional love and material support) is not true anymore: "Today one can have two, even three mothers, as the Tribunal of Rome wrote," in its decree on a case of surrogacy. These are the court's words:

> In the cases of surrogate motherhood the question of "who the mother is" cannot find an answer from a scientific point of view, as both subjects appear to be causally necessary to the process conducive to the birth; both women have a biological connection with the child. What is noteworthy, instead, is the problem of defining who will be the person having the duty to care for the newborn after delivery, and which of the two women should be considered socially responsible.[17]

But there is no ambiguity. The doubt and the confusion about exactly which figure is duplicated in this kind of ART stem from language, not from a supposedly essential modification of the biological process of procreation inaugurated by ART. Our languages have been forged over the ages in which the technical possibility of separating egg contribution and pregnancy was inexistent. The divisibility of these acts through ART has given rise to conceptual problems, as language does not change so easily, and the same word "mother" now stands also for a new concept: the egg contributor.

"Gestational surrogacy" (also called "full surrogacy") comes in two forms: either using the future social mother's egg or a donor's egg. Using an

---

[16] Or rather "became a zygote " Paola Tabet (2014, see also Martin 1991) questions the choice of words describing the embryo as a "fecundated egg," and with reason. This choice of language conveys passivity of the egg, as the feminine part that gets "fertilized" by the active sperm, the male agent, but in fact what happens is a fusion of the two gametes. This, argues Tabet, resonates with the attribution of fecundity only to women, as it is current in demographic discourse. In this case, I just wanted to highlight the vicissitude of the woman's egg.

[17] Tribunale di Roma, Ordinanza 17.2.2000.

egg from a woman other than the surrogate is a practice that has been developed over the last thirty years, and some say that it has now become the preferred one, as it can allow a couple to have a child that is genetically theirs. But the purpose for using donor eggs is to cut off the surrogate from claims of motherhood based on genetics, and purportedly even from her feelings, extolling DNA provenience over pregnancy.[18] In California gestational surrogacy seems to have nearly replaced traditional surrogacy, which was simpler both from the point of view of the technique and from the cultural consideration of the facts about motherhood. A lawyer working in Oakland with decades-long practice with surrogacy contracts affirms:

> The non-related surrogate is the general case now. Usually it is the donor's egg or the mother's egg, and the surrogate is not related: they call it gestational surrogate. This happens in 90% of the cases, the other 10% is what they call traditional surrogacy and the surrogate is officially inseminated in the doctor's office, usually. Then 1% is actually doing it at home, and there are financial reasons: they can't afford the IVF procedure. (Personal interview, January 2013)

Nevertheless the true proportions are unknown, though there are countries, as we will see, that mandate the gestational form in order for the agreements to be approved.[19]

From the material point of view, the (nonmonetary) price of the surplus of medical interventions to perform a gestational surrogacy is paid for by the surrogate mother, who submits to an unnecessary surgical operation to implant the embryo, and to avoidable but obligatory hormonal stimulation in the name of efficiency. From a contemporary cultural point of view, the lack of her genetic contribution tilts the balance of power in favor of the intended parents (whether the gametes come from their bodies or from a purchase) over the centrality of the pregnancy process in procreation. It is here that the true innovation lies, and it is cultural more than technical. The

---

[18] "When forced to acknowledge that women's genetic contribution is equal to men's genetic contribution, Western patriarchy could have foundered. But the central concept of patriarchy, the importance of the seed, was kept by extending it to women. Valuing the seed of women, the genetic material women also have, extends to women some of the privileges of patriarchy. That is, when the significance of woman's seed is acknowledged in her relationship with her children, women too have paternity rights in their children. [...] Children are, based on the seed, presumptively 'half his, half hers'- and might as well have grown in the backyard. Women do not gain their rights to their children in this society as mothers, but as father-equivalents, sources of seed" (Rothman 1989, 91-92).

[19] It is affirmed that 95% of the contracts in the US are for gestational surrogacy (Sanger 2007, 127 n.118).

first IVF with a "donated" egg and the consequent embryo transfer into the womb of another woman, did not create another "mother," the mother only by genes, but shifted the whole position of females in matter of procreation. A woman can now have the male experience of externally expecting a child that is genetically hers, if another woman bears the embryo derived from her egg. With IVF, women have assumed a role previously reserved to men, from gamete donation to the external wait. Of course there have always been similar situations: in adoption both the woman and the man wait "externally" for a child to come into their family, but the child is never genetically related to them. In surrogacy instead, for the first time since the beginning of the human species, there is the possibility for women to share the universal fathers' experience. An act of emancipation, perhaps, maybe even a step towards gender equality. But, more exactly, the emancipation from the "slavery of pregnancy" that Simone de Beauvoir dreamt about and Shulamith Firestone hoped for, is realized through the bodily engagement of another woman. As it stands now, the "barbaric act" (according to Firestone) cannot be entirely outsourced to machines—only to other women.

There is yet another concurrent for the title of "real mother," as the egg—as we have seen—can come from a third woman, a "donor," who contributes the genetic material in case the intended mother can't, and is generally not traceable. Of course this is the only possible way to proceed if the commissioning couple is gay. Lesbians seldom make recourse to surrogacy with an egg contributor, but it can happen.[20]

What place should we give to the egg donor? Aren't we disregarding her right to be called a mother, too? As she contributed the ovum, half of the DNA of the baby is hers, the baby will look like her, it will have familiar traits with her ancestors. But if we look at biological functions in gestational surrogacy, again what we have is not two mothers, but—as said—a woman taking on a male biological role: the gametes are coming from two "fathers," one male and the second female. And if the child will not visibly look like

---

[20] "Lesbian surrogacy" is a misnomer, sometimes used when a couple of women decide to split and mix their contributions to have a baby: one gives the ovum while the other undergoes the pregnancy, so both can have a biological connection to their child. Clinics rather call it "reciprocal in vitro fertilization," that is another misnomer. Some lesbian couples have tried to have their family recognized from birth in courts proving that one woman is the birth mother and the other a genetic contributor: it has worked in Israel in 2012, where the woman who donated an egg to her partner could become the second legal parent to their child (Shakargy 2013, 245).

the pregnant woman when both gametes come from others, her biological influence will be there because of the epigenetic process, of which I'll speak later.

So, when the genetic material comes from a woman other than the one who carries the baby, the role of this "mother by DNA," whose egg has been fecundated and transferred to the "surrogate," exactly replicates that of a father, so IVF and embryo transfer amount to a multiplication of *father* figures! Also the genetically unrelated intended mother waits externally, but her situation is closer to the intended mother in an adoption case (peculiarly created with her husband's sperm), while the egg donor does not wait at all. All these pretended "mothers" have nothing to do with what a mother has always done. But a concept must be expressed in language, and here words diverge from biology, deceiving us. As this "second father" is female, we must use the proper grammatical gender: I can't speak of a woman as "another father," everybody speaks of "another mother." Nevertheless the role of the genetic "mother"—until the baby is born—is still only to have contributed half of the genetic material, nothing more and nothing less. She is waiting like a father for a woman to deliver her genetically-related baby. Therefore conceptually she is not a mother: she has neither gotten pregnant, nor will she give birth—she is just a feminine father. It is only in grammar that the position of the mother and the one of the father are symmetric, distinguished only by their masculine or feminine gender. Jacques Lacan and Luce Irigaray wrote that language belongs to the Father, as it is the capacity to create and teach symbols pertinent to power, which in our society is male.[21] Maybe they were right, or maybe they have become right in the present cultural climate and disastrous consequences of the idea of gender equality applied to the wrong issues, even to biology. The grammatical gender symmetry combined with our idea of gender equality are only confusing the two very different biological roles of the male and the female. As said, this is valid only for the period of gestation: the genetic contributor can become a mother after the birth, as the social mother of the newborn.

In fact, neutral "parents" do not exist. The contemporary use of this neutral expression, besides muddling what mothers and fathers do in their

---

[21] When I talk and write about psychoanalysis I usually quote Meyer (2006). Despite the sensationalist title (*The black book of psychoanalysis*) it is a scholarly work, demonstrating the unusefulness and the damage of this nonscientific theory. But some good can always be found everywhere.

"parenting," has two more valid motives: one is a will to be inclusive of the many lesbians and the few gays that have children; the other is the acknowledgement of the appearance of "new dads," committed to rearing their children in what was previously considered a motherly way, that is without eschewing material care. Gay fathers are one prominent expression of this male desire to take care of kids. However rare "new dads" might be in reality, rarer still than same-sex couples with children, it is nevertheless a development in fathers' behavior much wished for by the mothers. According to Nancy Chodorow, the male entry in motherly care would also be useful to extol the material carer. The men who enter this "female" perspective will spread a positive view of human connections based on care, eradicating male ignorance and modifying their faith in the "autonomous individual."

IVF and embryo transfer do expand reproductive possibilities, in particular permitting a woman with blocked tubes (40% of cases of female infertility) to become pregnant by having her egg fecundated *in vitro*. And they have mixed up the biological sexes, as a future mother can now wait for her baby like a future father does, with no other biologically active role than the initial genetic contribution, while she helps and sustains her pregnant partner like a father should do. But it has surely brought confusion about who is who, in particular who is the "real mother." This confusion in turn has begotten undesirable consequences spilling over from the realm of surrogacy to our view of motherhood in general: the minimization and disregard for the role and contribution of the birth mother in this now decomposed process of making a baby.

But in fact, this is not new at all, as it mirrors the historical disregard of patriarchal societies for women's contribution to society in general, and to procreation (and subsequent care) in particular (Katz Rothman 2000). For example Aristotle believed and taught that the woman was only a receptical for the seed of the man, offering an environment in which the sperm would develop by itself. She was the dumb matter, he the smart form. She could therefore not have any claim to her progeny—it was really *his* progeny. This has served as an ideological basis for treating women as inferior beings, even in the biological act that is peculiar to them in its greatness, dangerousness and heroism: the bearing of babies.

Paola Tabet described how throughout history women's procreative powers have been devaluated as an object of exchange, to which women have been forced by male organized dominance. Women have been constantly denied the freedom and capacities of a true subject, their bodies put at men's disposal by male violence. Other second wave feminists—Phyllis Chesler, Janice Raymond, Carole Pateman—were adamant that in surrogacy the child was born to the father, as surrogacy helps when the intended mother is the infertile one in the couple. But they wrote before embryo transfer technology spread: if the infertile woman can nevertheless produce functional eggs, the child can be hers as well as his. Scathingly, Phyllis Chesler (1988) refers to the intended father as "the sperm donor" and Janice Raymond (1994) as "the ejaculator," completely denying his intention to become a father, and who in fact—together with the same will of the intended mother—must be credited for having started the whole process of pregnancy. The attempt to read the social process of surrogacy as a neat conflict between the sexes, with women lined up on one side and men on the other, has failed, as women have in a sense become more like men, in their public roles and also in reproduction. The fault line is not so easy to find now as it seemed in the '70s and the '80s, although the domination of families by men has not changed much.

But the participants in surrogacy have surely multiplied! To name all the people involved in the process I have used the most common denominations—the surrogate or surrogate mother, the intended parents, the donors—but the question of what to call all these people is not trivial.

Actors in the agreement

The first revolutionary act, said Rosa Luxemburg, is to tell the truth. When we call the woman who gets pregnant and gives birth to the child a "surrogate mother," we imply that she is not a real mother, she is just a substitute for the real thing. The journalist Katha Pollin suggested that she is more of a "surrogate wife."[22] "Surrogate" implies that she is not even quite up to the task, as "surrogate" is something that we can make use of, but as a second best: chicory for coffee, carob paste for chocolate, *I can't believe it's not butter!* for the original greasy product.

---

[22] Quoted by Krimmel 1992, 27). Original in Katha Pollitt, "Contracts and Apple Pie, The Strange Case of Baby M," *The Nation*, 682-84, 23.5.1987. See also Field 1988, 5.

By calling the pregnant woman "surrogate" all the dilemmas that I have described before about who the real mother is, appear to be easily solved: the woman who bears a child is just an aid, a helper, she does something that the real mother cannot do, but only on her behalf. She gets paid for it! Or she does it out of generosity, or—often at the beginning of surrogacy— because she is a member of the family and sees and shares the suffering of the childless couple. One of the first cases of implantation of an embryo not originated from the eggs of the surrogate herself happened in South Africa, where the mother of an infertile woman became the carrier of triplets generated *in vitro* with her daughter's and her son-in-law's gametes (Slabbert and Roodt 2013, 326).

This is what the language of "surrogacy" means: the *surrogate* will not be the real mother of the child, in the sense of becoming its social mother: this is a relationship that will be established between the intended mother (that is the *real* mother) and the child. In this denomination of "surrogate," the certainty of the termination of her role is implied. As soon as the baby is born, her help will not be needed any longer. She might have further contact with the child, but she will certainly not be a member of its immediate family.

The certainty of her disappearance from the scene is deceptive: as we will see in the third chapter, laws nearly everywhere in the world consider the woman who gives birth the legal mother. If surrogacy is not inscribed in other laws that contradict this fact, the uncertainty about who is going to raise the child will remain: the surrogate mother could decide to keep the child she gave birth to in a perfectly legal way. So "surrogate motherhood" is in reality mostly just an intention. But this is not the only instance of deceptive terminology in this matter, as lexical ambiguities, euphemisms, misnomers, and words that are used with a distorted meaning are mushrooming around surrogacy.

First of all, it is a misnomer to call "surrogate mother" the woman expecting the child, as a woman becomes a mother (any kind of mother!) only after the baby is born: there is no "mother of a fetus."

"Reimbursement of expenses" to the surrogate often includes a salary, under the disguise of "foregone gains" by women who are in fact mostly unemployed.

"Biological mother" is used for the intended mother who has given her egg, as in this phrase: "The biological parentage seems, thus, to be a solid support for the legal recognition of the maternity of the intended mother " (European Parliament 2013,136).[23] But besides the biological egg contribution, there is the contribution of pregnancy, and both are in terms of "biological material." But isn't the biological effort of the woman who bears and births the child a tad bigger than just giving an egg—however risky and painful the process of egg retrieving can be? By incorrectly equating the female biological contribution in gestational surrogacy only with her egg, the law of Illinois requires the impossible: "The gestational surrogate mother certifies that she is not the biological mother of the child, and that she is carrying the child for of [*sic*[24]] the intended parents."[25]

"Gamete donation" in practice almost never happens, as nearly all "donors" are paid. Sperm donation, practiced since the 19th century, started to spread in the '80s, with sperm sample requests for compensation appearing on the billboards of medical school faculties. It was an easy way for the young and careless to pocket some money, and it was done especially by medical students. The act was and is pleasurable, plus men aren't usually very concerned about whether their semen is going to generate another human being or not, anyway.[26] They could even consider it as getting some extra tickets at the genetic lottery to pass on their DNA.

Then came "egg donation," hardly comparable. Ova "donors," as said, can be the same women who undergo fertility treatments and who agree to leave the mature oocytes that they are not using to other women as this re-

---

[23] It is not a slip of the tongue but political strategy. This report to the European Parliament has been compiled by a group of lawyers and legal experts who find the contract the best possible configuration for surrogacy, using sympathetic language about the very few countries that have introduced its enforceability, while considering "backward" all other possibilities. They are clearly advocating the process of commodification of babies, as the above example demonstrates, and talk without doubt of a true parentage of the newborn by its intended parents: "It is difficult to predict the evolution of the jurisprudence even if there is a clear tendency in favour of the recognition of the child's parentage" (European Parliament 2013, 119).
[24] Interesting lapsus. The legislators could not really bring themselves together to clearly affirm that a child born from a woman is not hers.
[25] http://www.ilga.gov/legislation/ilcs/ilcs3.asp?ActID=2613&ChapterID=59   accessed 15..3.2015.
[26] Rene Almeling reports a funny anecdote: "when a new employee at Western Sperm Bank excitedly told a donor that a recipient had become pregnant with his samples, she said it was like 'somebody hit him with a huge ball in the middle of his head. He just went blank, and he was shocked.' During his next visit, the sperm donor explained, 'I didn't really think about the fact that there were gonna be pregnancies.' The donor manager described this state of mind as 'not uncommon'" (Almeling 2011, 78).

duces their bill at the clinics. So at least they will not be exposed to the risk of ovarian hyperstimulation, anesthesia and surgery just for the sake of it. In alternative, these women can be "donors" who get paid for each successful retrieval operation (not for eggs by the number) as the male sperm "donors" are. Unlike sperm donation, this opportunity to make some money comes with risks. Eggs do not come out so easily or pleasurably. The gains of male and female "donors" are hardly comparable, reflecting the respective inconvenience of the operations:

> thousands of dollars for the eggs and a mere fifty to one hundred for each sperm sample. The price list for ova varies with the general level of prices (reflecting the cost of labor) of each country, but also according to the personal characteristics of providers. The list is topped by the US where, despite the attempts of the American Society for Reproductive Medicine to set a "reimbursement limit" at 5,000 UDS, about 5–10,000 USD are offered, a sum appealing to all sorts of women in need and especially to students, as it more or less matches the cost of a year's college tuition. Students who have been admitted to Yale, Harvard or Princeton can get a higher price: they are offered 35,000 USD in ads in college magazines. Also Danish eggs can command more money, as they entail the promise of a blonde and blue-eyed baby (in Sweden and Norway egg donation has long been forbidden—in Sweden since 2002 only anonymous donation is—though women eager to make some money this way can go abroad to "donate"). Asian and black donors are in strong demand in the US, where their eggs are better paid than most of the whites'. Ukraine stands in the medium-range, with a significant difference: only 1,000 USD, lower than in Lebanon, where 3,000 USD are paid per cycle. Indian women are paid 100–300 USD per donation, and sometimes the "reimbursement" goes up to 500 USD. It is interesting that in the US sperm donation is easily conceptualized as a job, while egg donation is advertised as an act of giving: "In appealing to women's sense of altruism, physicians placed much more emphasis on egg donor motivations than they ever had with sperm donors. In fact, the earliest egg donation programs incorporated psychological evaluations, in part to assess women's motivations, again a form of screening that had rarely, if ever, been required of men donating sperm" (Almeling 2011, 36). Reproduction is allowed only to altruistic females: "'Girls who just want to lay their eggs for some quick cash' are rejected" (Almeling 2011, 59).

Hormones are copiously employed in a cocktail of artificially synthesized molecules that have the same effect as human hormones. They improve the overall risk/benefit rate: women mature only one egg at a time, occasionally two, while under hormonal hyperstimulation the number of eggs that mature can reach the number of forty. With hyperstimulation, generally between five and twenty-five oocytes become eggs and are accessed by aspiration inserting a needle guided by ultrasound into the belly. Since total anesthesia is needed (or other forms, but not just local numbing), it seems reasonable to get more than just one. That is, "reasonable" from the "overall" point of view. If we consider the point of view of the woman, she is made to run different kinds of risks: besides the anesthesia and surgery for egg retrieval, she submits to hormonal stimulation which brings pain and can cause ovarian hyperstimulation syndrome, other infections and bleeding, and eventual complications from surgery. Ovarian hyperstimulation syndrome (pain, abdominal inflammation, possible renal failure and infertility, venous thrombo-embolism and cardiac instability) has even, in rare cases, resulted in maiming and death.[27] In 1% of the cases the consequences of egg retrievals are classified as "serious" (for references see Almeling 2011, 4–5, quoting the American Society for Reproductive Medicine). And it should not be taken for granted that if only one egg is accessed the woman will necessarily repeat the operation. So, as usual, we see medical interventions multiplying on their own strength: it is never enough, and further manipulation is never avoided, as the first intervention rather legitimates all the subsequent. Once medical interference has started, it even appears that the more of it, the better the result must be (the C-section is considered simply the best, despite the increased risks to the health of the mother and the baby when delivery is not problematic).[28]

In conclusion, "ova contributors" or "egg providers" are much more accurate terms than "donors." And also their male counterpart should be named "sperm providers," as they never donate anything but—in sharp contrast with the rhetoric surrounding egg contributors—are clearly in it for the cash.

The usual denomination of "intended parents" seems the only correct name in the current terminology. Intention to become parents and arrangements for the pregnancy to take place, in fact, aptly characterize the infertile couple (or the individual) who want to become social parents. Nevertheless, those enthusiastic about surrogacy find that "intended parents" is inadequate

---

[27] It also seems that it enhances the risk of a mild form of ovarian cancer later in life: "Dutch researchers studied more than 19,000 women age 40 and younger who had I.V.F. and about 6,000 who had visited fertility clinics without having the procedure. After 15 years of follow-up, they found that women who had undergone I.V.F. were more than four times as likely than those who had not to develop borderline ovarian cancer, a malignancy that is treatable and survivable" (Bakalar 2011). The original study concludes with a call for further monitoring (van Leeuwen 2011, 1).
[28] The Slow Medicine movement is trying to change this attitude from within medical practice.

because eventually their intention becomes a fact.[29] This, as we have seen, should not be taken for granted. *How* exactly intended parenthood can become a fact is neither univocal nor uncontroversial.

The legal expert Yasmine Ergas is ironic about surrogacy terminology:

> In a model surrogacy contract, I recently saw the uterus-provider referred to as the "embryo-carrier." It's such a relief that we don't have to use the "M" word anymore! Nine months in the womb? That's not a mother, that's an embryo-carrier. Like the sherpas of colonial yore, she carries the embryo the way they bore the bags. (Ergas 2012a)

"Gestational carrier" is also used—but we can note that the expression "to carry a baby" is of common use, though not particularly respectful of the pregnant woman, who does not in fact only "carry."

Women themselves often describe what they are doing as "babysitting for nine months," or with similar self-descriptions: in chapter 4 we will analyze both the social representation and the self-representation of surrogate mothers. In this chapter I want to make sense of what happens by observing the facts.[30] A surrogate mother may declare that she is babysitting, but in fact she is the one who is materially creating the child, that is forming itself from her flesh and bone, with inconvenience and pain, for the duration of nine months in her womb, which is nothing more, nothing less than a part of herself. In fact, the most unacceptable terminology of all for surrogacy is the "renting of a womb," whereby women are made equivalent to only a part of their body. This choice of words equates the uterus to a thing (and also a baby to an artifact), but does not occur, as one might think, only in derogatory discourse. A Californian web advertisement read "Your oven, their

---

[29] Phyllis Chesler is also critical of this denomination for the opposite reason: "it is acceptable to restrict references to parenthood to the 'intended parents' as the other parties involved are only providers of either raw materials or services (in fact, surrogacy is the vehicle whereby the 'intended parents' realize their parenthood, which is what is 'intended,' presumably, by all the parties); finally, it is acceptable for all parties to engage in the transaction because it is not commercial and does not reify the children themselves as transactional objects (they are always-already the children of their intended parents)" (Chesler 1988, 16).

[30] I find useful the methodology described by Marvin Harris in *Cultural materialism* (1980), with the emic-etic distinction carried over from language studies to social analysis: it separates the point of view of the observer from the one of the observed, and ideas from behavioral facts, that scientific procedures always try to establish. All fields of studies are therefore legitimated, but with different meanings: studying ideas about social reality does not mean studying social reality as it happens, nor can it give reality its true—or better—meaning. See also the works of the Swedish anthropologist Alf Hornborg (e.g. 2001).

bun."³¹ This advertisement was of course aimed at intended parents, as they are the ones who are going to spend money with the clinics and the agencies offering these baking services.

Anyway, parts of the body like the uterus remain firmly attached to a woman—as in the German quip about the "Gastarbeiter" (guest-workers) that factory owners "invited" in the '50s: "We wanted arms, but whole people arrived." Moreover, the "guests," whom German entrepreneurs wanted to employ only during the economic upturn and then send home, did not intend to go back at all, bringing along their families instead.

So even if the original intention to have a baby did not come from the pregnant woman but from the intended parents, it was she who had the baby. She can feel and behave like the baby-sitter and "return" the child to the people she feels are its legitimate parents, but—during the pregnancy or after the birth—she could possibly, instead, feel that the baby is hers. Her joy and also her responsibility. Pregnancy in general does not always start with an intention, and sometimes the intention changes, as when two lovers split. Intention is not essential to conception, but in order to have a baby, gestation—that is the woman-fetus physical relationship—is.³² No matter how the "surrogate" feels, she *has* gone through the pregnancy, which is a factual relationship of dependency of the developing child on the mother's body.

Surrogate motherhood is essentially a relationship, not a matter of using things. The use of new reproductive technologies cannot cancel the persons involved. Many try to do so ideologically, but the facts are different, and the facts will not change until an artificial uterus is manufactured, a real oven to bake the baby in, an object producing human life from gametes (Bulletti et al. 2011).³³ If cheap enough it will be a good alternative to the

---

[31] Advertising banner at the top of the page www.allaboutsurrogacy.com (accessed 5.1.2013). An article sympathetic to commercial surrogacy by Agency 4 Solutions is entitled: "SUR-ROGACY: Your Bun, Her Oven...Is It Right For You?" 29.9. 2008 (http://community.barefootandpregnant.com/fertility/surrogacy_your_bun_her_ovenis_it_right_for_you/ accessed 19.12.2014).

[32] "Intent without biology contributes little to the creation of the objective entity known as a child" (Rae 1994, 100).

[33] Nearly half a century later, the invention of the artificial womb that Firestone envisioned has not yet been accomplished, despite attempts (a Japanese team for example works with acrylic and parts of living tissues). Yoshinori Kuwabara, chairman of the Department of Obstetrics and Gynecology at Juntendo University in Tokyo made headlines with his team's experiments with goats' fetuses (http://www.nytimes.com/1996/09/29/magazine/the-artificial-womb-is-born.html, accessed 18.12.2014).

complicated relationship of intended parents with a real woman carrying someone else's genetic child (or half-genetic child, or also not related at all).[34] In this case, money surely talks, and the baby will not be contended: the machine makes a product by its mechanical services. But who would dare to raise a child that has been borne by a machine? A human being that has developed the whole time inside a metal and plastic artifact? But perhaps, this child will be gifted, being much better "equipped" (or rather unequipped), to live the soul-less and self-destructive life of this late capitalist society.

In conclusion, "birth mother," a term I have already employed, must definitively be the best terminology for a "surrogate," because she is not a substitute at all. She becomes a mother the moment the baby is born. "Birth mother" is the denomination used in situations of adoption, it is a name that the "first mothers" of adopted children themselves are reclaiming, wanting to destroy the curtain of oblivion about the origin of adopted babies that authorities and mediators try to impose. So, though the situation of adoption is different, as the pregnancy that leads to it did not usually start with any intention, "birth mother" affirms the fact that a woman that has given birth *is* a mother, distinguishing her from the social mother. To keep calling a woman that gives birth a "mother" is not old-fashioned language: it is biology. To call her something different amounts to trying to ideologically deny what she has done—or rather "made" by nourishing, also emotionally, the fetus—and her paramount relationship to the newborn. She should not be forgotten, nobody should ever try to cancel her role.[35]

---

[34] Another possibility for infertile women that is currently being developed is a uterus transplant. The first baby from a transplanted womb was born in Sweden in September 2014. It had to be delivered prematurely, as the mother, a 36 year old woman born without uterus, had developed preeclampsia, possibly as an effect of the immunosuppressive treatment she had to avoid rejection of the new organ. The uterus came from a live donor, an older woman (Brännström et al. 2014, see also http://www.sciencedaily.com/releases/2014/10/141007092110.htm accessed 1.12.2014).

[35] "La madre dimenticata," Italian for "The forgotten mother" is the title of a short contribution that I wrote for *Orgoglio e pregiudizio* a booklet edited in 2010 by the feminist collective "Quaderni Viola" lead by Lidia Cirillo. The piece was censored and excluded from publication without even informing me, as "it showed only one side of the debate," as I came to know later. I haven't changed my mind since, and I believe that feminism is to be on women's side—in this case refusing to consider biological motherhood as something different from the physical gestational experience.

The possible alternative of "real mother" would be ambiguous, because of its current usage. Both birth and social mothers are real mothers. Adoptees sometimes denominate their birth mother in this way, but "real mother"—*a posteriori*—seems to be a much more apt term to designate the adopter, as in fact it is the social mother who has taken care of the children. She is not a "birth mother," but her rearing mustn't be disqualified.

Though there are affinities between adoption and surrogacy, in contemporary times "adopting" means finding parents for a child, while the surrogacy process centers exactly on the opposite: giving a child not yet existing to somebody who intends to be a parent. Adoption in rich countries is under strict rule and control by the state—not a bad thing, considering the conditions of "baby farms" in the past and also in contemporary poor countries. The transfer of parental rights cannot happen just by will and money: history has shown that this possibility creates markets for babies structured by economic agents that have a stake in the abandonment of the children. They re-sell the best specimens letting the others die (Balcom 2011).

Some lawyers have called surrogacy "the new adoption," as it permits skipping the queues for the fewer and fewer healthy babies relinquished, also (mostly) avoiding the requirements set for the would-be adopters or foster parents. In some places surrogacy also guarantees a more certain result, as in adoption birth mothers have a "change of heart" period, usually of several months, should they decide to rear their baby themselves.[36] Another overlapping feature of surrogacy and adoption is that in certain places, like the US and Greece,[37] the agreement can be reached during pregnancy: the adopters and the birth mother can meet, choose each other and draw up an agreement, that in any case must protect the right of the birth mother to keep on caring for her child if she wants. But also in surrogacy the outcome might not be—as originally agreed—that the social mother will be different from the birth mother, and that the mother's role will be taken over by the intended mother. It may instead happen that the tie between mother and child will not be severed by a birth mother who has also changed her mind. Is this change of mind and heart legitimate? Whom do the children belong

---

[36] Martha Field, who has written in 1988 an excellent book "dissecting" the surrogacy debate, proposes a cut off point much closer to the birth in cases of surrogacy, with no possibility for the birth mother to get the baby back once she has handed it over.
[37] Greek authorities have a nonchalant attitude to parent-child relationships: they take newborns away from *sans-papier* mothers, as they cannot legally recognize their children.

to, from a substantial point of view? (The legal point of view belongs to the next chapter.)

Second BIG question: Whom does a newborn belong to?

Let us go back to the conundrum of the "female father." The problem initiates from the fact that a woman, the genetic mother, nowadays can occupy a position that in the long past of our species only men could be in: her biological contribution to the new baby is solely genetic. But in terms of relationships with the embryo/fetus/developing child/newborn, she is a "female father" who does not have the biological experience of pregnancy and birth. That is, she becomes a mother in the social and not in the "natural" way.

I know that "Nature' is a difficult word to employ in an essay, as it is difficult to disentangle "Nature" and simply "what I prefer." Moreover, "Nature" is used by all kinds of ideologies, from various religions to sociobiology, to exemplify their preferred arrangement of society, or just to describe the status quo, thereby justifying existing power relations. "Nature" is also a difficult concept for our society, which believes that it has emancipated itself from Her.[38] Nevertheless I want to describe "the natural way" of becoming a mother as the act of getting pregnant and giving birth. It also implies a physiological, nonmedicalized process of delivery, as a normal pregnancy is not an illness.[39]

In talking about nature, I refer to the bodily activity and the experience arising from it. The division of sexes in nature has evolved in order to mix the genetic material in the procreation of some complex species, while others are genderless or hermaphroditic.[40] The very different task assigned to males and females can't be bypassed. The "pregnant man," Thomas Beatie, who gave birth in 2008 in the US, was born female, then transitioned to socially become male by taking hormones and subjecting himself to surgery to make his body as masculine as necessary to match his perception of himself.

---

[38] But Nature speaks for herself in my pamphlet *L'ecologia spiegata agli esseri umani* (Ecology explained to humans), available in Italian at www.danieladanna.it.
[39] For a discussion of "physiological" vs "natural" concepts of delivery, see Spandrio, Regalia and Bestetti 2014, 25 ff.
[40] Intersex individuals are also born in species with sexual reproduction.

He married a woman and they wanted kids, but she was infertile, so the couple decided that he would use his reproductive capacities in order to have a baby with an external sperm contribution: his uterus and ovaries were still intact, since their removal is not required to be recognized as a transsexual in all of the US states' law—a freedom that is fought for by transsexuals all over the world, who want the possibility to choose one's social gender without having to undergo either surgery or psychiatric control. The pregnancy occurred despite the fact that the male hormones he had been assuming for some time do influence pregnancy, though he had suspended them during it. The baby was born healthy.

This biological asymmetry cannot be treated under the general principle of equality between the sexes, as the contribution to procreation cannot be equal, and "nothing is more unjust than to share equally among unequals," as the school of Barbiana, guided by don Lorenzo Milani, wrote.[41]

The fact that the gender of the genetic-only contributors to reproduction is now changeable (only male or male plus female), has indeed the merit of clarifying that we cannot just speak about the prerogatives of the genetic mother. We must reflect on the broad subject of the role of a genetic contributor in relation to the baby. Is the genetic contributor (or "are the genetic contributors") entitled to become parents?

We can formulate the second BIG question like this: what rights should come with the genetic contribution that used to be only the father's? What to do socially about the genetic contributors to the conception of a child? Is genetic contribution enough to become a parent? Whom do the children belong to? The second BIG question can also be formulated with concepts specific to surrogacy: who gets to rear the child if the surrogate refuses to relinquish it to its intended parents? Who is entitled to decide who gets to rear the child? In sum: what is a family, what should a family be?

A first consideration is that there is no "birth father." At birth, but also during pregnancy, the genetic father could be anywhere doing all sorts of other things—or he could indeed maintain a close relationship with the future mother, and even be involved in delivery, physically and psychologically helping the woman in labor. He could also instead be unknown, or even—disgracefully—the child could have been conceived with an act of violence,

---

[41] The School of Barbiana: *Letter to a teacher* [1967], 31 (http://www.swaraj.org/shikshantar/LTAT_Final.pdf accessed 20.12.2014 accessed 2.10.2014).

with rape. This is also the reason why from the female point of view it is plainly wrong to affirm, as many say and write, that nowadays with the contraceptive pill "not only is sex possible without reproduction, but reproduction has become possible without sex" (note also that in this overused observation "sex" stands very restrictively for "coitus" alone). Sadly, reproduction has *always* been entirely possible without any sexual experience by the woman if she had been raped, as from the woman's point of view this is definitively not a sexual act. The *bon mot* reflects only the male experience of conception: coitus that ends with pleasure and orgasm. The female experience of conception has too often not entailed any sexual feeling, spanning from indifference to victimization.

The male genetic contributor to a new life becomes a father only by virtue of his relationship with the mother. If he is the husband, their relationship is officially recognized, conferring on him responsibility and authority over the children (and sometimes over his wife, as in the past). Marriage, to which the woman has consented, implies the future assumption of the father's role by her husband. *Pater est quem nuptiae demonstrant* (the father is the one indicated by marriage) in Roman law and in all marriages until the contemporary possibility of recognizing descendants first by blood samples (that could only exclude paternity, used since the '40s) and then by DNA analysis (which positively establishes it with near certainty, since the mid '80s) if a court so orders.[42]

In cases where there is no marriage, who decides what the family is going to be? Many legislations—all the codes derived from the Napoleonic Code—bestow the capacity to decide what the family is going to be on the single mother: the legal recognition of a child who is not yet 14 years old cannot occur without the consent of the "parent" who has already recognized the child. Despite the neutral legal language, this "parent" must always be the mother, as she is surely there with the child upon its birth, while the "father" cannot recognize something that is still in its mother's body and does not have a biologically independent existence, nor a legal one.[43] The

---

[42] In fact the possibility of anonymous parturition was given by the Napoleonic Code to avoid infanticide when the mother knew that the baby was a result of adultery.

[43] Anticipating the legal analyses of chapter 2, I'd like to quote a Dutch tribunal that in 2006 affirmed "that there was no close personal relationship between the man and the unborn child, since such a close personal relationship can only come into existence after the

mother thus has a priority right: she can refuse an unwanted recognition, or —on the contrary—she can request that biological paternity be recognized as legal against the will of the begetter of her child to obtain material support from him.

Marriage as a "reproductive contract" is increasingly refused by the new generations, who just cohabit. If an unmarried couple lives together, some countries consider it a common-law marriage, conferring on the cohabiting man the same prerogatives and duties towards the couple's children, or nearly the same, under the institution of "parental responsibility." Swedish law for example attributes the same status of a married couple to any couple, hetero or homosexual, living together, including responsibility over any minor who lives with them. In other countries an unmarried man must legally recognize the child as his own to be invested with fatherly duties and rights, and generally this must happen with the mother's consent (not necessary in French and Portuguese laws). Or the genetic father can be a friend, a fleeting relationship, a stranger, so if the pregnant woman does not want him in her family, he cannot interfere. Or he can be a donor, so he should likewise not interfere.

All this would be quite fine, but for a problem: courts are increasingly granting legal recognition of fatherhood against the single mother's will— and of course I am not talking of the thorny divorce cases where men did become fathers and took care of their genetic children, but of men who have contributed to the foundation of a family only with their sperm, and never had any significant contact with the newborn.[44] Even donors have been granted father's rights by courts validating their paternity suits (especially in the US). Unfortunately and unjustly, a mother's right to remain the sole parent is thereby limited. The presumed father can sue to obtain recog-

---

child's birth" (Vonk 2010, 140, summing up Rechtbank Assen, 15 June 2006, LJN AY7247).

[44] Barbara Katz Rothman identifies the importance given to genetic contribution with patriarchy itself: "This is the ultimate meaning of patriarchy for mothers: Seeds are precious. Mothers are fungible. Today we are more familiar with the nonbiological services that we hire from mother-substitutes. We hire baby-sitters, day-care workers, nannies, housekeepers, to 'watch' our children. The tasks are the traditional tasks of mothering - feeding, tending, caring, the whole bundle of social and psychological and physical tasks involved in the care of young children. When performed by mothers, we call this mothering. When performed by fathers, we have sometimes called it fathering, sometimes parenting, sometimes helping the mother. When performed by hired hands, we called it unskilled" (Katz Rothman 1989, 97). She rightly advocates for visitation rights of sacked baby-sitters.

nition of his fatherhood by a court regardless of the mother's will, arguing that the recognition would be "in the child's best interest," as this principle is also mentioned in family law and international conventions. This rather empty concept[45]—tentative at best, as it refers to the future development of an infant and of its family relationships—is increasingly interpreted by courts to be equal to "having a father." But the primary interest of the child should instead be recognized as growing up in a stable and nonconflictual environment, not with family ties imposed by a court. With whom then should the child be placed if the surrogacy agreement is not respected? The mother or the father, that is, the intended parent(s)? Must it depend on their respective wealth? Psychological stability? Attitude to "parenthood"? Can experts really forecast which of the two environments will be stable and which would be the best for that particular child?

No. Neither courts nor experts should be entitled to decide how a family is composed. The family already exists, and it is based on the Mother/Child relationship. If we recognize the relationship between mother and child and put it at the centre of our concept of the family instead of the sexual relationship between men and women, we no longer regard the family as the product of the sexual act (an imprecise concept if the woman has been forced to sex and if the parents are lesbians or gay). In terms of relationships, a family at birth looks different. The only recognizable social relationship is based on the biological fact of pregnancy: the expecting woman and her future child are the basic form of family, at its minimum. And the best interest of the child, its well-being, is to have this relationship recognized as its minimal familial unit (besides it, of course, mothers are always imbricated in a web of social relations: motherhood never happens in a vacuum). The best interest of the mother is to be entitled to a relationship that starts in her womb, and then to be able to allow (or not) other adults into this relationship. Or even to renounce this tie with the child if she really so wishes. Therefore culture and law should change their current positioning that defines the "best interest of the child" as having a mother and a father. The

---

[45] This is admitted by Jean Zermatten (2010, 485), Director of the International Institute for the Rights of the Child and Vice-Chairperson of the United Nations Committee for the Rights of the Child: "If we analyse the best interest principle as a whole, there is no particular explanation of its application. It does not outline any particular duties, nor does it state precise rules," as every child is different. Then he admits that what is applied are the theories most in vogue (see also Fineman 1991, proposing the primary-caretaker rule).

mother, the whole woman with her virtues and defects, is indispensable to the birth and the natural nourishment of the child,[46] who cannot really choose her, as it wouldn't be in the world without her choice.[47] But the father must be chosen by the woman: through marriage, through other kinds of covenants, "changing gender" by entering a lesbian relationship, even relinquishing the child to "intended parents" biologically related. She might be wrong, the man she chooses might not be the best possible father for her offspring, but she is entitled to choose this relationship, as she is entitled to make her own errors in her life. It would be an act of violence by the courts to impose on her a familial relationship with a man that she does not want, even if he is the genetic father of her child. It would also be an attack on the well-being of the child, who must start life in a "family" already broken, as it is plainly absurd to impose a family life on two adults who do not agree on being together. The father's (imposed) rights means in fact that the infant will be carried back and forth between two homes—as (luckily!) courts cannot impose the sharing of a home on the generating couple. But not necessarily will the legal parents collaborate: tensions, quarrels, fights can erupt between them following the rights that the court ordered to be shared. Joint custody, the arrangement increasingly imposed to affirm the ideological equivalence of the two "parents" in the children's upbringing,[48] would surely be out of place where the father is unknown to the newborn. Other kinds of custody, which according to a legal dictionary encompasses the care, control, guardianship, and maintenance of a child, are definitively out of place, too. Visitation rights also limit a mother's decisions about who should have access to her child. Contact upon reaching a certain age, if requested by the

---

[46] I agree with Stephanie Lynn-Budin (2011, 91) that "all association between children and women after the cessation of breast feeding (or, following Bolen, parturition) are entirely cultural," adding that breast-feeding, which is undoubtedly better for children in a normal situation, must also be a woman's choice and right (See also Katz 2000).

[47] An Irish verdict recites: "Under Irish law the 'natural mother' is given automatic guardianship and a personal right to custody of the child under Article 40 of the Constitution. As guardian the mother retains full responsibility for the child unless this is permanently removed by an adoption order. She is presumed to act in the best interest of the child and the court is reluctant to intervene" (Harding 2013, 225).

[48] Fineman comments the international trend of joint custody based on a misapplied equality principle: "Custody policy at divorce reflect the determination that parents are assumed equally entitled to custody regardless of the 'mothering' they did (or did not do) during the marriage." (Fineman 1995, 71). In Italy legal recognition as father of a newborn was granted to an ex boyfriend whom the mother denounced for domestic violence (Danna 2009, 127-130).

child and agreed upon by the genetic contributor, is the only possible specification of the rights of the genetic contributors, as all legal authority over the child must clearly rest with its mother. This is also in the best interest of the child because, if there is such a right as a birthright, it must mean at its minimum to enjoy a stable and peaceful environment, even if this means to grow up "without a father"—or more exactly, without the genetic father, while the social role will probably be assumed by a present or future partner of the mother. Phyllis Chesler clearly traced the parallel between surrogacy and custody cases:

> Baby M is every child who has ever been physically, legally, or psychologically separated from her birth mother "for her own good" in the mistaken belief that a child needs a father, a father-dominated family, and/or money far more than she needs her birth mother, love, and freedom. (Chesler 1988, 17)

To grow up without a father does not necessarily mean lacking the male role model, as it can be found in the extended family or among friends. Even if there is no father figure in the cohabiting family, a child usually grows up with a plurality of adults among which a fatherly figure can be chosen, if the mother feels that it is beneficial for the child, who by the way will increasingly be able to express itself and its needs.[49]

So much for the totally unclear concept of a child's "best interest," that has become a fetish to impose its separation from its birth mother in surrogacy (even creating a catch 22 situation: "How could a good mother agree [have agreed] to give up her child?" rhetorically asks Kelly Oliver 1989, 100). This unsubstantiated criterion has been used in Italy to overthrow the relationship criterion, even in cases of infants, in the name of the social conformism of having a father and a mother—although in different homes!

The question of the presence vs. absence of a father is current, as formal marriage is less and less practiced, while couples separate often, and cases of separation during pregnancy are not unheard of at all. What has been shown by social research is that a large quota of the separated fathers distance themselves from their kids. The father's role is often taken up by a new partner of the mother:

---

[49] It is understood that if the parental powers to which a child is subject are misused, the state should and will intervene with its social services on behalf of it. But in the normal upbringing, children are dependent on their parents' choices by definition.

In the US, in fact, after a divorce, 40 to 50% of children lose contact with their fathers. In France, it was already estimated at the end of 1985 that out of the 2 million children living separated from their fathers, 600,000 no longer met with them. In Denmark, another research conducted in the '80s found that 20% of the children did not have any contact with their fathers anymore. (Pocar and Ronfani 2008[3], 214)

In Italy during the '90s, one third of the children had no contact after separation or divorce (Barbagli and Saraceno 1998). Men—under present conditions—do not always show a very strong interest in their relationship with their progeny. Care work for the children is mainly performed by mothers, as time-use surveys worldwide show (e.g. Eurostat 2004, Folbre and Nelson 2000), so the relationship between mothers and children is stronger than between children and their fathers. The "need for a father" is often intended by psychologists as intervention of a third person breaking the mother-child tie. This social role represents larger commitments: it is the authority symbolizing the necessities of life in society. This role can easily be performed by a woman, and in fact there is often a polarization of the two mothers in a lesbian couple: one with an affective-permissive role and one with more impersonal rule-giving tasks. But in this debate, many speak of a "male role" consciously having in mind the traditional male—on which I have extensively written in Italian, so I can now quote Martha Fineman in English instead:

> Socially "appropriate" male gender behaviour is often characterized by feminists and others as punitive, repressive, and dismissive of women. Men, either as fathers or as sons, might more appropriately be concerned with how we might act as a society to change this dominant imagery of masculinity. If fathers fail to challenge the violent and misogynist aspects of the culture, a question might arise as to what is the purpose, or point of providing them access to children? (Fineman 1995, 206)

But many feel that genetics and intention should prevail on the mother/child family tie. History unfolds in curious ways. Genetic fathers, who have historically used "intention"—or rather, their lack thereof—to deny women they made pregnant their care and support for the ensuing child, now want to use "intention" as the one and only parameter to attribute parental responsibility when surrogacy agreements fail. When women fought for a right to sue for judicial declarations of paternity forcing men who got them pregnant to marry them, their aim was to get material support from "runaway fathers," in order to maintain a social status that the life as a single mother would have destroyed. The Napoleonic Code did not admit paternity suits precisely in order to protect "wealthy and inexperienced youth" who could be dragged into fatherhood and its disbursements "by fallen women without scruples."[50] Nevertheless a paternity suit can still be what the mother wants, trying to obtain material help or to win back an ex-lover through his responsibility for the infant. The Italian jurist Ines Corti comments on this:

> The will to procreate is not decisive in matters of paternity attribution—but this again is not an absolute principle, rather one tied to social circumstances: its basis is the protection of the mother who suffers from social and economic problems in absence of a father, so if she wants the natural father to share his responsibility in procreation (not having used contraceptive devices), then society supports her claim. From this an absolute principle of truth in matter of procreation does not descend. (Corti 2000, 210)

Here the proposal of Fineman for collectively contributing to the rearing of children could cast a different, less legitimate light on this claim. But on the contrary now in the US and in the UK the state tries to identify the genetic fathers or the new boyfriends of single mothers in order to impose on them the financial burden that the languishing public sector of this neoliberal era does not want to shoulder anymore.

When single women in the past wanted their babies to have a father by turning to courts, heterosexual social relationships were marked by homosociality, and the family was mainly an economic and productive unit. Therefore it made sense, economically and socially, to force an unwilling man into marriage—marriage was in any case often arranged and even imposed by the older generation. Scant attention was given to the quality of sentimental relationships in choosing a lifemate. As women started to be more economically independent, family relationships changed, and love marriages with reciprocal feelings came to be preferred. But until quite recently the legal status of being married trumped any true will of the spouses whether to be sexual with each other, so a man could pressure an unwilling woman to marry him. He could then rape his wife, as she would be legally obliged to have sexual relations with him, all this coming under the concept of conjugal duty. Great masterpieces of 19th century literature have described these attempts: don Rodrigo tries to marry Lucia against her will in *I promessi sposi* by Alessandro Manzoni, and the Comte de Guiche tries to force Roxane first to marry a complacent man and then himself in *Cyrano de Bergerac* by Edmond Rostand.

---

[50] *Relazione al progetto preliminare del Libro I* [of the Italian civil code], quoted by Alessandro P. Scarso, in *Trattato di diritto delle successioni e donazioni*, Giuffré 2009, edited by Giovanni Bondini, p. 286. In the exquisite original Italian, it was the worry that: "giovani inesperti e doviziosi" would be chased after by "donne perdute e senza scrupoli."

This is the world that "we have lost" (luckily, I'd say). The women's revolution in the 20th century extolled the importance of being true to one's feelings, and to live feminine lives that are free from coercion in intimate relationships: marital rape has been denounced as a crime by women's movements, and the CEDAW has spread this notion around the world, helping local battles: now marital rape is outlawed in most countries. The concept of a family based on bonds of affection is prevailing, and the law should finally recognize it.

Chapter 2)
From conception to the baby

Fertilization and the beginning of pregnancy

Texts dealing with surrogate motherhood—mine included—usually start with the explanation of the difference between traditional and gestational surrogacy, and they also stop there. The adjective is explained, while the noun is taken for granted. But what is motherhood? What is conception, what is pregnancy, what is delivery?

In order to comprehend the process of surrogacy, and in order to sweep away any doubt that still might be hovering about who the mother is, I find it important to describe the biological developments and processes in becoming a mother in the flesh. Not because it should be substantively different in surrogate agreements from all the other kinds of pregnancies, but because—before proceeding to analyze both the law on surrogacy and the cultural consideration of it by its participants—we must be sure to know what we are talking about. Absurd definitions abound in literature and conversation. One example is the expression of sympathy for the insurmountable pain and sorrow that the intended parents would suffer if the birth mother decides to break the agreement and keep her baby: "They have been waiting for the child, they have been expecting it for nine months!" The pregnant woman did not, of course. Not much value is given to the experience of the biological mother, while the intended parents are pitied, as for nine months they should live in uncertainty—which is by the way intrinsic to the process of pregnancy in many other ways. But intended parents have a typical White, middle-class vision of the procreative process: voluntaristic, manageable, supported by technology and an essential vehicle of happiness, as Zsuzsa Berend concluded in her 2010 analysis of the forum www.surromomonline.com.

Coitus or artificial insemination at the proper time, determined by the woman with self-observation of her menstrual cycle, start the process of surrogacy. Artificial insemination can be performed without the manipulation of the seminal fluid and gametes, in a sort of natural way. But generally this is not how it is done: insemination takes place under the control of doctors in a clinic, where sperm is manipulated and the woman who tries to become pregnant must first assume hormones to regulate her cycle and enhance her chances.

The principle followed is that "Doctor knows best," while Nature can always be improved upon. This is called "the technological ideology" by Katz Rothman. Acceleration is another principle ruling innumerable aspects of contemporary society, geared to reach an "economic optimum" of (apparent) efficiency. And once unpleasant procedures are in place, nobody wants to submit to them multiple times. Money is a factor, too. The more efficient the pregnancy rate per cycle of insemination, the better for its consumers, as each attempt is pricey and only few countries include ART in the common health care of their citizens.

So, hormones are used *en masse*. This is an example of a protocol in a clinic:

> Start BCP's 3–4 days after the start of your cycle
> Start Lapron 14 days after the start of your next cycle
> Start Estrace 7 days after your cycle
> Lining [of the uterus] check between 6–7 days after start of estrace
> Transfer up to 14 days later
>
> A breakdown of the meds for that cycle (before transfer)
>
> 33 BCP's
> 28 Lupron Shots
> 20 Doxycycline Pills AM &PM
> 8 days of Vivelle patches (ranging from 1 @a time to 2 @a time)
> 16 asprin pills
> 6 Medrol Pills
> 21 estrace pills
> 1 Valium
> 5 PIO IM Shots
> 2 Progesterone Suppositories
> Prenatal vitamins for the entire cycle (Alexander 2006, 51)

The protocol of the clinic is undisputable:

> One of the questions you should ask the R.E. [reproductive endocrinologist] during the initial visit is—how long does your clinic require me to continue meds once the pregnancy is established? Not all clinics will give you a straight answer about their protocol,[51] but as with any other question you've asked thus far—you never know until you ask. According to the online surrogacy message boards, there have been reports of some surrogates who were required to continue meds until 8 weeks of pregnancy and others who continued until 14 weeks of pregnancy or longer.
> Asking these questions earlier on will help prepare you not only physically but mentally.[52] (Alexander 2006, 64)

But, preparation aside, problems can always arise:

> any procedures might create future problems with conception: "fertility" treatments could render a fertile woman subfertile [...] If a woman knew the certain psychological stress and likely physical harm in IVF, could she ask any other woman to help produce her baby? How could physicians carry out such schemes—even if their priority was to alleviate suffering of the childless? Is this "healing"? Or is it a spell cast by technology and by pleas of potential patients? (Bequaert Holmes 1986, 49)

Current procedures in a clinic involve concentration of the sperm by elimination of most of its seminal fluid, in order to place it directly in the uterus, which would otherwise reject it. The sperm is put into a culture, and will be centrifugated to obtain gametes in a concentrated form. Sperm are then put with a little pipe into the vagina or the tubes (if the clinic believes a little more than usual in natural processes), or into the uterus, or also used for in vitro fecundation with ripe eggs that must be harvested, after the now familiar "controlled ovarian hyperstimulation." In vitro fertilization of eggs and sperm can occur simply by putting them in contact, or by the more interventionist injection of chromosomes directly into the egg nucleus. This ICSI (intracytoplasmic sperm injection) is done in case of "weak" sperm. Many steps in the natural fusion of the gametes (still unknown to scientists) are

---

[51] This resembles the situation in India, where surrogates are *never* told about medical issues: "The surrogates interviewed at both the sites commented frequently on the medication regimen that was prescribed for them. Since most of them were not informed of this prior to their decision to enter into the arrangement, and because often assurances were made that the surrogacy pregnancy would be like their earlier ones, surrogates had no idea about the levels of medication they were required to take; this was not something that they had considered at the time of entering into the arrangement" (Sama 2012, 80).

[52] Latashia Alexander's instructions to fellow surrogates show her belief, spread in the US, in the power of rational prevision to program one's feelings, even in dramatic circumstances: "*Who will hold the baby(ies) first?* As some IP's would want the child passed to them first, you need to be on the same page regarding where the baby(ies) will go after, make sure that you know beforehand so that there are no hurt feelings in the end" (Alexander 2006, 77).

skipped by using this injection. The current image of the egg patiently and passively waiting for the winner of the sperm race to penetrate it, is completely wrong. The egg captures a sperm, interacts biochemically with its particles, and actively modifies its covering and its structure before the fusion of the two DNA chains.

The obtained morula is then put in a Petri dish, waiting for it to multiply its cells, until they become eight in few days. Two of these cells are often removed for a genetic analysis. As for all other kinds of genetic and gamete manipulation, the long-term consequences of this practice are unknown and unresearched, though it seems that everything is fine, as a new and complete human life does grow out of the six cells left. The embryos are observed, eliminating the abnormal ones. The embryo transfer to the womb is made 2–4 days after the fecundation, by means of a catheter, and anesthesia is not required. As seen, the woman has usually been given hormones, starting weeks before the transfer. She must keep on self-injecting them daily, up to a couple of months, as they enhance the possibility for the zygote to nest, avoiding miscarriages. They harmonize the menstrual cycle of surrogate and intended mother, whose eggs are extracted and fecundated in vitro. The surrogate's own maturation of eggs must be stopped in order to be able to receive a zygote derived from another woman's egg.

And this is what happens "Before and after the transfer," related by Latashia Alexander:

> Before the transfer commences, you may or may not be given a Valium pill to relax during the procedure. Usually performed 3 to 5 days following the egg retrieval, during this procedure you may be required to have a mildly full bladder so that your uterus can be seen by abdominal sonogram during the procedure. Usually the attire will be a hospital gown and no clothes from waist down. Next, you will be instructed to lie on the table with your legs in stirrups. The RE [reproductive endocrinologist] will then insert a speculum into the vagina and clean the cervix. As with a pap smear, you may feel cramping as an outer catheter is placed through the cervix into the lower segment of the uterus. A small catheter is then placed though an outer transfer catheter and advanced near the top of the uterus. Once the placement is correct, the embryos will be expelled from the catheter and inserted into the uterus.
> After the transfer is complete, you will go into the recovery room where you will be instructed to rest on your back for at least two hours. (Alexander 2006, 53)

In order to guarantee nesting in the uterus, multiple embryos are used at one time. The flip side is that all of them might nest, starting a multiple pregnancy which is much more dangerous than carrying and birthing a singleton, both for the mother and for the developing children: preeclampsia and gestational diabetes for the pregnant woman, preterm and/or operative delivery are the risks enhanced by multiple gestations.

Nevertheless, following the principles delineated before, it seems reasonable to try to implant more embryos to improve the success rate, reducing the time, money and stress involved on all parts—especially on the woman who tries to become pregnant. But who takes these decisions? This is peculiar to the different clinics, only a few national laws deal with this matter.[53] It is also a matter of where the power lies: surrogates in India do not have any other say after volunteering to become pregnant, as Sama (Resource Group for Women and Health), the Centre for Social Research, Amrita Pande, Kalindi Vora, Usha Rengachary Smerdon and other researchers have shown. The doctors take all the decisions, and even volunteering is often a family resolution to which women obediently submit—as we will see in chapter 4.

When multiple embryos nest in the uterus, to avoid the perils for the health of mother and children, and to avoid having to care for more babies than wanted, another technique is deployed, called "embryo reduction." It consists of aborting one (or more) embryo(s) that appear less healthy, while sex selection should be forbidden. This can only happen in countries where abortion is legal:[54]

> SD2, who had yet to deliver the child in her second surrogacy, had already been approached by the agent for entering into a third arrangement in which the commissioning parents' demand for a male child would be accommodated by sending SD2 to Thailand, where the surrogate would undergo a sex-detection test and consequently a sex-selective abortion, towards bypassing the impediments of the legal framework in India. (Sama 2012, 67)

The decision about this procedure is not a technical one, but it is in fact one of the greatest conflict points of surrogacy, as we will see.

---

[53] See the *One at a time* webpage: http://www.oneatatime.org.uk/372.htm (accessed 20.12.2014).
[54] Unfortunately not everywhere, despite the CEDAW recognized the reproductive right to access to safe procedures to interrupt a pregnancy, when the pregnant woman does not accept the life conceived. The embryo is inextricably connected to her body, it is still not a separate being, so it is the woman that can and must choose whether to care for and nourish it or separate it from her womb interrupting the pregnancy.

The "pregnancy results"

Using a sexual relationship for achieving fecundation is not a very widespread method, as the intended parents are usually a monogamous couple, and the "surrogate" usually has a monogamic partner, too. Artificial insemination, *in vivo* or *in vitro*, is nearly always used. How successful these techniques are, depends on a variety of factors. One of them is the fitness of the gamete providers and of the birth mother herself. Ova coming from an aging woman have less possibility to become viable embryos. The International Committee Monitoring Assisted Reproductive Technologies, a board of specialists, found that IVF and ICSI (inserting the DNA from the sperm directly into the egg) were both successful in one case in five, while the subsequent Frozen Embryo Transfer (FET)[55] is successful only in one case out of six: "The overall delivery rate per fresh aspiration for IVF and ICSI was 20.2% compared with 16.6% per FET" (Sullivan et al 2013, 1375). Embryo transfer resulting in pregnancy and delivery ranges from a success rate of 31% in some clinics, down to 9% in others, according to the report summarizing the most wide-ranged and recent collection of data on all forms of ART in 2,184 clinics from 52 reporting countries and regions (but still related related to the year 2004). Hope and faith in assisted reproduction techniques are constantly spreading, no matter how disappointing the success rate is—though this should also be considered in the light of the low success rate of intercourse in human reproduction: our species is not a very fertile one.

Multiple pregnancies and deliveries, albeit reduced, are still a big proportion of ART pregnancies: "The overall proportion of deliveries with twins and triplets from IVF and ICSI was 25.1 and 1.8%, respectively, but varied widely by country and region." Premature delivery is high, too: "The proportion of premature deliveries per fresh aspiration for IVF and ICSI was 33.7% compared with 26.3% per FET." The following datum is difficult to compare with the absolute perinatal death rate, as it is a synthesis comprising different regions of the world with very different health conditions to start with: "The perinatal death rate was 25.8 per 1000 births for fresh as-

---

[55] Embryo freezing is employed in cases of non synchronization of cycles, or if the same woman is subject to egg retrieval and implant, as the hormones used for egg retrieval do not favor pregnancy.

piration for IVF and ICSI compared with 14.2 per 1000 births per FET" (in Italy it is 7–9 per 1,000).

Longitudinal observations (the monitoring started in 2004) show that the procedures for ICSI and embryo transfer are growing in proportion: they are mainly used to bypass problems of sperm "weakness." It has also become more common to transfer fewer embryos, also because of authorities' interventions:

> Notably, the increasing proportion of cycles that are FET, the change in practice to single embryo transfer and the cessation of the transfer of three or more embryos in some countries has resulted in improved perinatal outcomes with minimal impact on pregnancy rates. (Sullivan et al 2013, 1375)

The disadvantages in the health of the babies born with the help of ART are well known and also documented in the report: "Higher incidences of congenital anomalies and of both autosomal and sex chromosome abnormalities specifically have been reported in both IVF and ICSI compared with spontaneously conceived infants" (Sullivan et al 2013, 1388). That ART babies are somehow disadvantaged in terms of health, is to be expected because of the very nature of ART, which make the infertile fertile, often using their own chromosomes and bodies: "It is difficult to determine the degree to which these associations are specifically related to the ART procedures versus any underlying factors within the couple, such as coexisting maternal disease, the cause of infertility, or differences in behavioral risk (eg, smoking)." (ACOG 2005). Some research[56] did not find any difference in the health of ART babies:

> Most retrospective and prospective follow-up studies of children born as a result of ART have provided evidence for congenital malformation rates similar to those reported in the general population. In contrast, an Australian study of 4,916 women found that the risk of one or more major birth defects in infants conceived with ART was twice the expected rate (8.6% for ICSI and 9.0% for IVF, compared with 4.2% in the general population). As with other studies, the control group was not ideal because it did not include couples with infertility who conceived without ART. (ACOG 2005)

This is possible, as the medical definition of infertility is that procreation has not been achieved by the couple after a certain period of attempts, that experts have diminished over time from two to one year. The conclusion of

---

[56] See original text for the numerous references.

the report is that more studies are needed to further define the risk of ART to offspring, which does exist.

From the implanted embryo, the future baby develops. The embryonal phase ends at the eighth week, then the fetal phase starts. This stage is the one in which the growing organism gets its arms and feet, and the facial feature characteristics of our species appear, differentiating the human fetus from the other mammals. Senses develop. Tact becomes functional already towards three and a half months; the sense of hearing after the sixth month; smell develops at six or seven months; taste at around seven-eight months; and finally the sight, which takes more time: the infant won't be able to see at its maximum potential before the age of three.

As its senses develop, the fetus' cognition of the pregnant woman's body and of her activities and relations develop as well. The future mother's body is the most immediate environment that surrounds the fetus before the birth, and information is absorbed from it as well as from the larger environment in which she lives, and from the people she interacts with. If its genetic parent(s) are not in the presence of the future birth mother, the developing child does not possess even a vague cognition of them.

And the pregnant woman's body is not a passive environment at all! Aristoteles was wrong—even apart from genetics—because the mothers' body influences the embryo and then the fetus through material exchanges. This is called epigenetics, that is "what happens around the genes," especially in terms of the hormonal makeup. Hormonal messages modify the structure of the embryo, contributing to its unique mental capacities, illness-resistance, neurological structure, and other physical features (remember the controversy about hormones making male fetuses gay). In comparison with genetics, epigenetics is the Cinderella of contemporary thought: in vulgarized science all is attributed to DNA, giving people a sense of ineluctability, as if everything in social life had been anticipated by our genes. Epigenetics, on the contrary, speaks about the influences of the environment on the developing child—primarily the maternal body but also the whole of the environmental stimuli and substances absorbed or perceived through her belly: sounds, temperature, presence of particular elements in the air, the water and the food that the future mother takes in.[57]

---

[57] And also her stress. Field (1988, 89 ff.) quotes work by Melvin Zax, Monika Lukesch, Gerhard Rottmann, Peter Hepper, Brent Logan and many others, on the effect on the

A difference is there between surrogacy and other pregnancies: surrogates report to distance themselves mentally from the developing child. They do not talk to it, nor touch it very often, leaving these activities to the intended parents. The developing child is imagined as a very unwelcome guest, and five months of its fetal movements are ignored (Teman 2010, 75 ff.).

Delivery and detachment

Between the 37th and the 42nd week pregnancy comes to term, and birth approaches. Does the "industrial delivery," as many call the normal birthing process in developed countries, have something to do with how we have ended up even considering the possibility of having a baby, and then taking or leaving it by contract? Indeed, the impersonal way in which births occur in our society does not seem at all unconnected to the idea of women being used—and volunteering their bodies—as machines to obtain babies. This social attitude trivializing procreation does not start of course at delivery: the whole antenatal care by its specialists has been developed in order to control women's bodies during pregnancy, while the efficacy of its philosophy of treating all pregnancies as potentially abnormal is questionable. Ann Oakely wrote:

> When antenatal care began, a few per cent of pregnant women were regarded as "at risk" of their own or their fetuses' mortality and morbidity. The task of antenatal care was to screen a population of basically normal pregnant women in order to pick up the few who were at risk of disease or death. Today the situation is reversed, and the object of antenatal care is to screen a population suffering from the pathology of pregnancy for the few women who are normal enough to give birth with the minimum of midwifery attention (Oakley 1986², 213)

The woman in labor who enters a hospital's or a clinic's birth department, will most likely be admitted to a Goffman-style total institution that uses rituals such as the relinquishment of personal clothes, a tricotomy, an enema, to mark her body as property of doctors. After these questionable procedures, the lower half of her body will be considered 'sterilized," that is, out of reach for anybody who is not a health professional working there.[58] She is

---

well-being of the newborn and on the learning capacities of the fetus of stress, the desire to have a child, and other factors active during pregnancy.
[58] But we are constituted of a human body and a myriad of bacteria, that the mother passes over even to the fetus before birth (Gilbert 2014).

in a strange environment, under surveillance, more in the company of machines than of people. In the labor room her waters get routinely broken. As the woman in labor reaches the second stage of delivery, she will be put in the recumbent position and at this point she will have to submit to another painful ritual: an episiotomy. She will be attached to a fetal monitoring machine and a drip-feed apparatus, her veins perfused with synthetic oxytocin to accelerate the dilatation. At this point, to shoulder the increased pain from the oxytocin (contractions become instantly stronger) she will for sure ask for an epidural anesthesia that lessens her ability to feel her body and push the child out. The fact that women ask for epidurals is fully understandable in this context. The tolerance of pain, that gives the possibility of pushing more effectively by feeling the contractions, and eventually of experimenting the descent of the baby through the birth channel as pleasurable, can only happen in a supportive environment, that women certainly cannot obtain in the hospitalized birth, with intimidating, downright frightening conditions.

Though there have been attempts to invert the course,[59] the fear about something that should be a natural process is pervasive, as the institutions where births take place do not reassure women. On the contrary: they organize the work of the medical personnel as if they were on an assembly line, with babies obtained as "products" at its end. Personnel chat during the woman's labor, infantilize her, operate on her body as if she were an object without explaining the procedures, without asking for her consent, disrespecting to the highest degree this unique moment in a woman's life.

An excellent study on how the "assembly-line delivery" is conducted took place in the '80s in Milan, Italy (Regalia, Colombo, Pizzini 1984). Participant observation of 106 deliveries took place in five different hospitals and clinics, each with its particular birthing style—one was offering a "humanized delivery," that was little different from the others. All verbal and physical interaction of all people entering and exiting the waiting and the delivery rooms were recorded, and their spatial positioning as well. Impersonal

---

[59] The COST network "Building Intrapartum Research Through Health - an interdisciplinary whole system approach to understanding and contextualising physiological labour and birth (BIRTH)" is calling attention to the best practices. I thank Ramon Escuriet Peiro, Claudia Meier Magistretti, Eleni Hadjigeorgiou, Ema Hresanova, Mário Santos, Irene Maffi, Deirdre Daly, Josefina Goberna Tricas, Sigfríður Inga Karlsdóttir who have kindly sent me updated information on delivery practices.

and depersonalizing practices, barely masked as "scientific procedures," were thereby unveiled: they were in fact aimed at expropriating women from their centrality in labor, turning them into passive objects of medical manoeuvres and chemical inducement:[60]

> Sometimes, and this happens everywhere, the visit [in the labor room] is also associated with a manual operation to enlarge the edges of the cervix in order to accelerate the dilation. This happens more if the woman is considered "troublesome." It is to this kind of woman that the procedures for acceleration are often addressed.
>
> [From the field notes] The doctor examines the woman and says to the midwife: "Yes, she is giving birth, there is still a bit of rim but you can almost take her in" (into the delivery room)—the examination continues. Woman. "Ouch" (screaming).
> Doctor. "You mustn't say ouch. If you want to be helped, push towards my fingers and please keep your mouth shut."
>
> This maneuver seems to be performed off the record, because the staff makes no confirmation, even to colleagues, of having done it, nor it is recorded on the woman's clinical chart.
>
> A doctor is examining the woman who suddenly shouts: "That hurts!" - The nearby midwife casts a look of reproach at the doctor and says, "Hey, what are you doing?"
>
> Doctor. "Nothing."
>
> Later, the midwife declares "that guy has a heavy hand, and who knows what he's capable of doing to get it over fast."
> The personnel present there realizes that manual dilation is being performed by the evident reaction of pain by the woman in labor, not warned at all about what they are about to do. (Colombo and Regalia 1985, 73)

Sheer brutality was exposed in the practice of the obligatory cutting to enlarge the vaginal opening. The consequent stitching up was also performed without anesthesia (apart from the worst cases), scolding the women who expressed their pain. The same brutality plus scolding happened during the routine, again mostly unnecessary, of carving up of the uterus in search for the remains of the placenta, without even checking first whether it already came out intact.

I cannot help but compare these offences to the awe that people are encouraged to feel during the rituals of all religions. The men's words get

---

[60] Ann Oakley wrote in the same year that: "The possible hazards of induction of labour, even using the most up-to-date technologies, include iatrogenic prematurity, and increased use of other interventions (e.g. epidural analgesia), fetal distress (as a result of oxytocin stimulation), neonatal jaundice, greater labour pain and unhappiness in the mother resulting from her passive role in the delivery of her baby" (Oakley 1986, 207). This is still confirmed today (e.g. Spandrio, Regalia and Bestetti 2014).

worshipped in churches, mosques, temples, but the women's unique deeds (or words, for that matter) are trivialized and trampled upon.[61]

Unsurprisingly, satisfaction is low:

> In Cartwright's study, 81 per cent of the 2,378 surveyed mothers wanted to be able to exercise choice about the medical management of their pregnancies and labours. Seventy-eight per cent of women who had their labours induced, did not wish to repeat the experience, but 93 per cent who had their babies spontaneously would choose to do so again. (Oakley 1986, 208)[62]

This hasn't changed, nor stopped (McIntosh 2012, Spandrio, Regalia and Bestetti 2014). "I will not have a second child," tells me a friend, the mother of a one year old girl, who gave birth to her in an Italian hospital.

Dehumanization has already occurred. Women in the birthing process have been deprived of their own timing, strength, capacity, to be put on an industrial assembly line. Franca Pizzini comments: "The generating power of women has been harnessed by technology; it is no longer able to scare men, who have the science, and the knowledge to apply it" (Pizzini 1985, 136). Then she quotes Chadeyron:

> The woman is depersonalized, she must be silent and stay still. She is an embarrassing container through which one comes into contact with the fetus. Obstetricians monitor the baby inside the woman, who is considered inconvenient [...] The pregnant woman is far less than a sick individual: she is nothing more than the container of the fetal object explored by technology. (Pizzini 1985, 136)[63]

This "development," that has rendered the woman in labor a simple passive object on which doctors act to extract a baby, is akin to thinking that making a baby and delivering it to somebody else should be an easy act, feasible even on behalf of total strangers, or even a job.[64] What is most astounding is

---

[61] For an imaginative contrast, see the description of the Palace of Birth in the dystopic novel *Egalia's Daughters. A satire of the sexes*, by Gerd Brantenberg (The Journeymen Press, London 1985, Norwegian original 1977).

[62] Original reference: A. Cartwright: *The dignity of labour? A study of childbearing and induction*, London, Tavistock 1979, p. 107.

[63] Original quotation in Chadeyron P.A., *La machine et l'obstetricien*, in *Ginecologia psicosomatica & psicoprofilassi ostetrica : evoluzione e prospettive. Atti del 1. Congresso congiunto delle Società italiana e francese di psicoprofilassi ostetrica. Venezia, maggio 1976*, edited by R. Cerutti. Piccin, Padova 1976.

[64] But the story of Kim Cotton, the first "surrogate mother" in the UK points in fact to the opposite (Cotton and Winn 1986): She had delivered her first child in an hospital in the mid-'70s and was so horrified by the experience that for her second baby she insisted on having a home birth, mostly uncommon at that time. She recalls that it was so unusual that 3-4 obstetricians wanted to assist her. But when she volunteered to be a surrogate,

that these very strange conceptions are typically shared both by intended parents and by surrogate mothers, as we will see.

But let us now assume that the mother has had the best physiological delivery, in the positions that she has chosen, that her words and wishes have been carefully listened to, her requests fulfilled by the "birth team" of her choice. Let us also assume that the newborn is not narcotized as result of the anesthetics given or requested by the woman during labor.[65] What happens then?

The newborn is able to recognize its mother (her voice, her smell), and finds comfort in her physical proximity. It is reciprocal: the mother is pleased by the presence of her newborn, her level of oxytocin peaks in the meeting of the two protagonists of the birth. This meeting is nowadays recognized as one of the stages of delivery, because of its hormonal effects. Instinctively the newborn knows that the mother is its source of nourishment. They have known each other long before birth, as even the infamous Report on surrogacy made to the European Parliament recognizes:

> It has been well documented that important biological bonds[66] are developed during pregnancy. The odour of an infant is attractive to the mother, while sight and skin to skin contact further promote psychological and physiological bonding as important hormones like oxytocin are in operation. Surrogacy interrupts the process of bonding that starts during gestation and continues after birth and this is a very important reason why many surrogates refuse to relinquish the child. (European Parliament 2013, quoting Tieu 2009)

---

she underwrote an agreement with an obligatory hospital delivery, wrongly supposed to be safer. Israeli surrogates, for whom surrogacy is a job, mostly choose a C-section fearing to emotionally bond with the baby at birth (Teman 2010).

[65] Reality is different, as it has been denounced since the '70s: "Then we are administered all kinds of drugs, very often against our will, and must spend our energy on the delivery table turning away from persistent offerings of gas. Our movements and choice of position are restricted, and we are most often forced to deliver strapped down to the modern cold, hard delivery table which instinctively feels too high from the floor. And then after a delivery including numerous potent drugs, perhaps the use of forceps and a compulsory episiotomy, our child is taken from us to be observed by strangers in a nursery full of screaming babies. At this point, if the mother is undrugged, she is overwhelmed by maternal feelings. She wants to examine, touch and hold this baby she has waited so long to see. Instead the baby is detached from the sounds, smells, tastes and closeness that are her/his birthright. The father often gets his first look though a pane of glass. Where is there room for love? How can mother, father, and child share the true bond of these moments so vital to their mutual growth?" (Frediani 1982).

[66] But the "bonding theory," an analogy to the imprint process in some other species, is discredited. See *Mother-Infant Bonding: A Scientific Fiction* by Diane E. Eyer (1992).

Immediately after birth, the newborn reaches for a nipple, and when she or he suckles for the first time, the mother responds with an hormonal reaction that makes it easier for the placenta to detach itself (this could even happen in a hospital, should the personnel allow it). Judith Lothian describes their first meeting on the website of the World Health Organization:

> With her baby in her arms, the mother is engrossed, excited, at peace, proud, and astounded at the miracle she has produced. No one tells her what to do. They know that *she* knows what to do—not because she and her baby have read the books or attended Lamaze class, but because their journey has physically and emotionally prepared them both for this moment. The weight of her baby on her belly helps her uterus contract and expel the placenta. Baby stays warm in his [*sic!*] mother's arms. Baby knows just what to do to survive in the world he has entered. He is awake and looks around. Within seconds or minutes, he has his hands in his mouth and is smacking his lips. Unpressured, he slowly but methodically crawls to his mother's breast and self-attaches. As he nurses, his mother's uterus contracts, insuring that bleeding will not be excessive. The two greet each other unhurried, confident, and unpressured. Together, over the next hours and days, they will get to know each other and fall in love. (Lothian 2000)

Or maybe not. In cases of surrogacy, this depends on the will of the mother, but generally also on what has been agreed upon by the mother long before birth, before even getting pregnant. Maybe her will is not paramount anymore. The agreement—in some strange places protected by the law as a contract—must specify if the mother is going to have the baby in her arms at birth, if she will feed it, if her milk will be accessed and bottle-given by the (ex-intended) parents, how often they will see each other again. Can this agreement be respected? Must it be?

The woman made a promise. The baby that she bore is now alive and kicking, and admittedly it would not be there if the pregnancy did not start with the very intention of separating child and birth mother. Can she do it? What will happen in the delivery room? Who will act? Is she pressured to relinquish the baby? What does she really want? What about the reassurance of the newborn by maternal presence? What about mother's milk? It is all in the agreement. But can she really act like a machine that delivers a product? In fact this is how she has been treated during the whole process starting from "antenatal care" to the final stitching up: women have been expropriated of their birthing power. Women are all taught to be just a fetal container to be acted upon.⁶⁷ Surrogacy is only one extreme, where the women themselves fully embrace this vision.

If the birth mother relinquishes her baby, what will she think and feel after having complied with the agreement? She has severed the ties that the newborn has developed with the only part of the world that s/he knows—her body, voice, physiological rhythms—what is the child's reaction going to be? Will it miss her? For how long? Babies forget, the pain—or just discomfort—will go away. But again—without wanting to generalize some perhaps very peculiar situations—some babies can't calm down if kept away from their birth mother. A birth mother who fought to keep her baby appears in the documentary *Breeders* by Jennifer Lahl (2014). Heather says that her daughter, a very pacific baby during the first days together with her, after having been taken into the care of the intended parents could not be calmed down for months (see chapter 3). And of course it is well known from the popular press that Zac, the child of Elton John and his husband, spent his first five months desperately crying. (According to the press, the music star and his husband had the idea of trying to calm him down by fetching his mother's milk daily from 10,000 miles away by their private jet. It did not help.)

But of course newborns are flexible, they must be. They will adapt to the new circumstances. They will grow and make up their own minds about the procedure that brought them into the world, into a particular family. As adults, some of the "surrogacy babies" are already campaigning in order to be able to know their birth mothers, as a part of the movement of young people who have been generated with a donor's contribution and want to know their genetic parents, organizing "Anonymous father's day" and demanding the legal possibility of anonymity to end. They might be a tiny minority among all people "born this way," but they do exist.

What about the birth mother? The original "birth mothers" on the other hand, are the women who chose this name to define themselves: they gave up their babies for adoption but now are fighting to see them again. They also fight against the "adoption industry," both private agencies and social services, that fosters it by persuading women to give up their newborns, which young mothers usually do in order to get back to their teenage

---

67 In casual meetings with strangers, pregnant women get routinely admonished, advised, and of course scolded by strangers (The VOICE Group 2014).

lives—and/or for economic reasons. This transaction is minimized, too, by agencies, doctors, social workers, and lawyers, who do not recognize the difficulty in breaking the mother-child relationship and the possible future regret. Claude, one of these birth mothers, keeps a well-known blog where she writes about her experience and her fight, hoping to discourage young women from making the same choice that she did, and to avoid the continuous pain and regret this has caused her.[68] She writes me:

> One of my earliest "online" friends was a surrogate, so I have always seen a direct correlation between a surrogacy situation and adoption relinquishment. I strongly believe the same long term risks apply to surrogacy and the children will likewise be affected like the adoptee now. If anything the whole assisted reproduction industry has completely ignored all the evidence from adoption and they have literally NO excuse for making the errors they are with humanity. But if anything they have seen what has "worked" in adoption and used the worst to make surrogacy work. For instance the whole "family builders" mindset of a "good deed" taken on by a surro is a version of a birthmother kool aide on steroids. That said, there does seem to be a distinction within the surro community and they do NOT align themselves often with birth-mothers.[69]

The situation is certainly different, as many more birth mothers in adoption than in surrogacy regret it. The team led by Susan Golombok, director of the Centre for Family Research at the University of Cambridge found no damage to the psychological health of surrogates followed for ten years after their experience (Jadva et al. 2003, Golombok and Murray 2003, MacCallum et al. 2003, Golombok et al. 2004, 2006, 2011, Imrie et al. 2012, Jadva et al 2012). But regret does exist for a minority. There are still no systematic studies on possible long-term effects of this experience on the children, but the Cambridge team found more adjustment problems of 7-year-olds born out of a surrogacy agreement (when they know it) than in those born from donated eggs and sperm—clearly not a definitive result given the precocious age of the subjects (Golombok et al. 2013). For intended parents, in addition to the insecurities common to all gestations, one point must be added: to obtain a child in a guaranteed way from this process and agreement is only possible if a law affirms that the mother of the child is not the woman who bore it. Now is the moment for the law to make its appearance.

---

[68] http://www.adoptionbirthmothers.com/musings-of-the-lame-an-adoption-blog/ accessed 10.1.2015.
[69] E-mail correspondence, 9.12.2014, on file with author and with permission to quote.

Chapter 3)
Baby and the law

From status to contract

The passage from "status" to "contract," seen as the epitome of progressive and liberating modernity, was first theorized by Henry Maine, who described this aspect of the rise of the bourgeoisie in detail. Promoting its own material interests, the third estate subverted the social order that had unjustly divided human beings into rigid status groups. Is this same liberating passage from status to contract now including parenthood? In fact, surrogacy prospects the dissolution of 'mother" as status, transforming it into a contract. Many commentators, especially legal experts, hail this possible development as a liberation, for individuals will now be able to *choose* their own destiny also in matters of parenthood (with the paid help of lawyers themselves). Is it "progress" or is it merely the progressive commercialization of everything that Karl Marx and Friedrich Engels forecasted as the result of expanding capitalist forces of production, now also involved in the arrangement of reproduction, for the infertile but potentially for anybody? Who will buy parenthood, and who'll be bought, if this transformation takes place?

Another historical trend in capitalism is abstraction in defining the social notion of property. The establishment of a register for land, ever more precisely measured, enabled the buying and selling of portions of territory based only on an abstract ownership title, without respect for any actual engagement with the land. It certainly freed the concept of property from all material action: capitalism turned real property into pure will (backed up by state violence) detached from material possession, from cultivation or any other kind of soil exploitation, not to mention simply inhabiting the land and getting resources from it by gathering and hunting, as aboriginal peoples did in vast areas before European colonization. In fact, the system of "title by registration" (Torrens system) was first experimented in the periphery: applied in Australia from the mid-19th century on, only later was it imported to the center of the British empire with the 1925 Law of Property Act (Bhandar 2015). Moreover, the right of the proprietor was, at least at its beginning, unbound: he could do with land and nature whatever he wanted, including destroying natural habitats, polluting them and—of course—displacing aboriginal inhabitants.

As it happened with property, an abstract concept of parenthood is being introduced in law, too, and with the same purpose of easing its commodification. As land can be bought and sold without much more than exchanging papers, children will be assigned to "intended parents," disregarding the will and feelings of the birth mothers, and pretending to cancel the relationship that they have by the simple prior signing of a contract (backed up by state violence). The money the "surrogate mother"—and especially all intermediaries—receive in exchange will silence all opposition. It is a controlled sum, recalling the beads and bottles of spirit offered to indigenous people to buy "their" land, for which they had no property concept.[70]

For these changes to take place, in order for intended parents to be recognized as such even before birth and even without any genetic connection, just by buying eggs and sperm from selected "donors," new legal creations are needed. The universal principle *mater semper certa est*—the mother is the one who gives birth—stands in the way of attributing parenthood by genetics or even by mere intention. In this sense, in fact, legislation generally forbids not the practice of surrogacy, as we have seen, but the disposal of the mother's *status* with a contract before the woman actually becomes a mother. *Mater semper certa est* can be waived only by the woman herself in cases of anonymous delivery, with her final decision taken after birth—that is, after having become a mother—during a reflection period. The principle *mater semper certa est* appears in international conventions, such as the European Convention on the Legal Status of Children Born out of Wedlock (1975) signed by the Council of Europe member states: "Maternal affiliation of every child born out of wedlock shall be based solely on the fact of the birth of the child" (art. 2). In cases of litigation over surrogacy, before the diffusion of the gestational variety, courts of various countries have generally applied this principle. This is the synthesis of an early German case:

---

[70] In her book about the Baby M case, Phyllis Chesler unmasks the political role of the "experts" and of the ideology of "civilization" itself: "according to the mental-health experts, Mary Beth could do no right. They used everything she said and did against her, they disapproved of her *because* she had bonded with Baby M—as if this proved that she was no better than an animal. It's as if these experts were nineteenth-century missionaries and Mary Beth a particularly stubborn native who refused to convert to Christianity, and what's more, refused to let them plunder her natural resources—not without a fight" (Chesler 1988, 26).

Oberlandesgericht (OLG) Hamm, 2nd of December 1985, 11 W 18/85 (*FamRZ* 1986, 159; *JZ* 1986, 441; *NJW* 986, 781): A woman having had the role of surrogate, with the agreement of her husband, was inseminated with the sperm of another man. The child was born, and the surrogate and her husband refused to give him/her to the intended parents. The court declared that the fact that the mother concluded a surrogacy convention is not sufficient reason to separate the child from her, as the fact of separating a child from the family where he/she was born is an exceptional measure, taking place only when a physical or mental injury in relation to his/her wellbeing is observed. (European Parliament 2013, 112)

In the '80s, the surrogacy "contract" was proposed and signed in a number of countries as a way of fixing, freezing the pre-pregnancy intentions, but if brought to court they were generally invalidated as entailing the sale of a child. For example, in the Baby M case the motivations for declaring it void were that:

> The surrogacy contract conflicts with: 1) laws prohibiting the use of money in connection with adoptions; 2) law requiring proof of parental unfitness or abandonment before termination of parental rights is ordered or an adoption is granted; and 3) laws that make surrender of custody and consent to adoption revocable in private placement adoptions. [...]
> The surrogacy contract guarantees permanent separation of the child from one of its natural parents. Our policy, however, has long been that to the extent possible, children should remain with and be brought up by both of their natural parents. [...]
> The whole purpose and effect of the surrogacy contract was to give the father the exclusive right to the child by destroying the rights of the mother. [...]
> This is the sale of a child, or, at the very least, the sale of a mother's right to her child, the only mitigating factor being that one of the purchasers is the father. (In re Baby M, 537 A.2d 1227, 109 N.J. 396—N.J. 02/03/1988)

The change of heart by the US courts took only a few years, and it happened when gestational surrogacy took central stage. The technological novelty of embryo transfer made the issue look entirely different, and genetic mothers could appropriate children in even an easier way than genetic fathers. When two mothers—one a traditional surrogate, the other a gestational one—broke their agreements, the judiciary treated the cases in a completely different way. In 1988, as we have seen, *In re Baby M* a recognition of the birth mother was decided, but in 1993 in *Johnson v. Calvert* it was affirmed that the genetic provenience of the ovum plus intention to procreate made the baby belong to the genetic mother, while the birth mother was declared "not a natural mother."[71] But also the first case, the famous dispute between Mary

---

[71] The case was rather complicated: "Unfortunately, relations deteriorated between the two sides. Mark [the intended father] learned that Anna [the gestational surrogate] had not dis-

Beth Whitehead and William and Elizabeth Stern, turned out to be very negative for the birth mother: Baby M was placed with her intended parents. The birth mother had asked for custody but obtained only visitation rights. The principle applied was the "best interest of the child," and the Sterns seemed more stable and were surely more financially wealthy than the Whiteheads.

So the "best interest of the child" argument used by the Court had the practical effect of partially validating the contract, assuring custody to the father and his wife. It is strange that there should be any question about what the best interest of a newborn is, because it is obviously to continue the only relationship that it uninterruptedly has had until its birth with its mother.[72] But this was considered open to various interpretations of the present and speculation on the future. (By the way, the Sterns divorced, but how could the jury have possibly divined it?) The "best interest of the child" appeared internationally first in 1989 in the UN Convention for the Right of the Child: "In all actions concerning children, whether undertaken by public or private social welfare institutions, courts of law, administrative authorities or legislative bodies, the best interests of the child shall be a primary consideration" (art. 3.1). This very elastic criterion has had classist, racist and homophobic interpretations, as the juries and their experts presume to be able to know the future development of a child in different family configurations and compare it. This is an impossible task.

The best interest of the child was again necessary to privilege the privileged in *Johnson v Calvert* in 1993 because the Court could not bring themselves together to declare that the birth mother should be separated from her child, even if not genetically related. The court looked up the *McGraw-Hill Dictionary of Scientific and Technical Terms* and found that a new organism was the product of two gametes, none of which belonged to Anna Johnson. But she did not lose her child due to the blood-test evidence, nor to the

---

closed she had suffered several stillbirths and miscarriages. Anna felt Mark and Crispina [the intended parents] did not do enough to obtain the required insurance policy. She also felt abandoned during an onset of premature labor in June" (*Johnson v. Calvert*).

[72] Some legal experts—but not many—recognize it: "As far as the child is concerned, she [the mother who gives birth] is the only mother that he or she has had any relationship with. The intending mother/child connection exists only in her mind, and in that sense, it is a one-way relationship. It is difficult to see how there can be a relationship that could not possibly be acknowledged by one of the parties in the relationship" (Rae 1994, 99).

contract declared "legal and enforceable," because the court also decreed a prohibition of specific performance:

> But the court will not compel performance of all contract obligations. For instance, even when a party to a contract for personal services (such as employment) has willfully breached the contract, the courts will not order specific enforcement of an obligation to perform that personal service. Just as children are not the intellectual property of their parents, neither are they the personal property of anyone, and their delivery cannot be ordered as a contract remedy on the same terms that a court would, for example, order a breaching party to deliver a truckload of nuts and bolts. (*Johnson v. Calvert*, 851 P.2d 776—Cal. 1993).

The case was sent back to the lower court to decide custody and visitation on the basis of the "best interest of the child," and at this point Anna Johnson lost. It remained unsaid in the verdict, but as she was a Black woman working for White and Asian intended parents, in no way would she be allowed to raise "their" child. This verdict of the California Supreme Court opened the doors to the establishment of an internationally renowned surrogacy industry. In the verdict the male point of view on procreation, which does not entail the pregnancy experience, triumphed while the two "mothers" were pitted against each other:

> We conclude that although the Act recognizes both genetic consanguinity and giving birth as means of establishing a mother and child relationship, when the two means do not coincide in one woman, she who intended to procreate the child—that is, she who intended to bring about the birth of a child that she intended to raise as her own—is the natural mother under California law. (*Johnson v. Calvert*, 851 P.2d 776—Cal. 1993)

Some writers in favor of contracts were not happy with this double argument for the recognition of parenthood that also considered paramount the intention to procreate. They would have preferred genetic proof alone:

> This application of contract principles to family relations was both inappropriate and unnecessary. (…) the Court could have held that maternity, like paternity, requires a genetic relationship between parent and child. (…) it relies on the most important connection between a mother and child as the determining factor of motherhood. (Place 1994, see also Shultz 1990)

Obviously the fact that "the most important connection" between mother and child is genetic, reflects the experience of male procreation (not male social parenthood), which supposes also in motherhood, as is evident for many in fatherhood, a difference if the gestated child is genetically related or not:

> This [The Greek law that admits the validity of contracts only for gestational surrogacy] is based on the rule that for a woman to be forced to relinquish a child, with whom she has not only a gestational but also a biological [*sic*, intending "genetic"] bond, is excessively limiting, and, therefore, socially, morally and legally intolerable. If this would be permissible by law, it would have been contrary to the general principle of fairness and social ethos (art. 179 GCC [Greek Civil Code]), and would render the agreement invalid on the basis that it was immoral. (European Parliament 2013, 288)

And now courts and laws in general draw the line between traditional and gestational surrogacy by not forcing genetic mothers to relinquish their child. But the line drawn at gestational surrogacy in fact turns the gestational surrogate mother into a legal breeder.

This change of heart of the courts occurred in Italy, too: the first judiciary case involving surrogacy dates back to 1989. The woman "contracted" was a young Algerian, and the intended parents sued her because she refused to relinquish the child after birth in order to extract more money from the couple, who had already given her the promised 15 million lire (a little less than 10,000 dollars). The jury's decision was that the surrogacy contract did not comply with "public order:" it was judged to be on a par with the sale of children, and it did not matter whether the exchange of money was for a good cause—most certainly not to raise a slave for the house as in ancient times.[73] But in the year 2000, the Tribunal of Rome deliberated just the opposite in a case of gestational surrogacy. A woman born without a womb had a clinic produce and freeze embryos from her eggs and her husband's sperm. Only four years later did they find a suitable surrogate, or "donor," as the judge called her, in the person of a friend of the couple. In the meantime a Code of conduct had been approved by the Italian doctors' professional order, forbidding all kinds of surrogacy (it was 1995, and in 2004 a law on ART confirmed the prohibition). The couple asked the Tribunal for a green light to the clinic to implant the embryos, as their agreement preceded the adoption of the code. It was the only way for them to have a child genetically theirs, as the frozen embryos would deteriorate after five years.

The judge argued that, since "superincubators" starting and finishing a pregnancy were the object of research, it would be wrong to attribute the

---

[73] In the US (and elsewhere) markets in babies should be against the law even if children are not viewed as commodities by the buyers: "However the fact remains that [in surrogacy] children are still being bought and sold, something that is inherently immoral and in violation of the Thirteenth Amendment, irrespective of the surrounding circumstances" (Rae 1994, 51).

status of "mother" to the pregnant woman: "the gestational mother has an accessory and 'interchangeable' function, as she could, as hinted above, in a future that does not seem so far, be substituted by technological devices."[74] With this science-fiction reasoning, he authorized the clinic to implant the embryos (though he did it also because there was no commercial use of the friend's womb but just the "loan of an organ"). He went on to criticize the Italian Civil Code based on *mater semper certa est*, as not being up to date with the new technologies (yet to come... maybe...):

> In the surrogacy contract there is a problem concerning the unavailability of status, to which the hypothetical object of this court proceedings—the simple gestational motherhood—is irrelevant, as it occurs when a woman only brings to term with gestation an embryo resulting from the fusion of the spermatic material [*sic!*] of the commissioning couple, therefore genetically unrelated to her.

By letting herself be inseminated under contract, the judge reasoned, the carrier had abdicated her parental role.

Another verdict was delivered in 2008 in China against a mother by contract who had taken back her child by the People's Court of Jiangnan District, Nanning City. The court had to decide about a contract that Chinese law had already explicitly prohibited back in 2001. But, as in the Baby M case, the "best interest of the child" was used to take the child away from his mother:

> The trial judge held that:
> a) The surrogacy agreement between the plaintiff and the defendants was null and void, as it manifestly violated Chinese public policy;
> b) Under the Chinese Marriage Act, both the father and the mother have custody of the child; and
> c) The issue of which parent the child should reside with shall be determined in accordance with the best interest of the child.
>
> The judge went on to reason that in the present case, awarding custody to the Zhao [the intended parents] conformed to the best interests of the boy for the following reasons. First, Chen had entered into a commercial surrogacy contract voluntarily and transferred custody of the boy to the Zhaos after delivering the baby; and on the other hand, suffering from infertility, the Zhaos signed a contract with Chen, the surrogate mother, to have a child [paying her 150,000 yuan], and they exercised custody after the boy was born. Though the surrogacy contract per se was null and void, the above facts demonstrated that the Zhaos had a stronger intent to have and raise the child. Secondly, Chen was an unemployed girl who lived in a poor and remote village, whereas the Zhaos had a stable, high income and lived in Nanning, the capital of Guangxi Zhuang Autono-

---

[74] Tribunale civile di Roma, sez XI, 14 febbraio 2000, giudice C. Schettini *Contratto in genere. Contratto di sostituzione di maternità in determinati casi. Validità* (http://www.diritto.it/sentenze/magistratord/roma14_02_2000.html accessed 20.12.2014).

mous Region: therefore the Zhaos had an obvious advantage in terms of economic status. Hence the Court awarded custody of the boy to the Zhaos on a "best interest of the child" analysis. (Huo 2013, 98–99)

So much for the "People's" Republic. Notwithstanding the fact that Chen was also the genetic mother, the baby was taken away from her because of economic motives, and the surrogacy agreement, supposed to be void, was also given some consideration. The story as reported does not mention any visitation rights for her. The surrogacy contract is therefore exerting a growing influence—as is the commodification of everything, which we call globalization—also on the country with the second GDP (that is production measured by money) in the world, the possible future hegemon of the capitalist world-economy.

Both Carmel Shalev and Paola Tabet consider this movement from mother's status to contract as positive, but from very different angles. Shalev finds that women, to be considered equal to men, must be able to enter into a contract to offer reproductive services, and accept being punished for not fulfilling it by being forcibly separated from the newborn, lest they be considered deprived of rationality and driven only by hormones[75]—the arguments used in the 19th century to justify women's legal inferiority.[76] She never mentions the question of the relationship between mother and newborn—in fact she likens the work of a pregnant woman to the creative work of a sculptor, that has an object as a result. She also does not acknowledge that from the 19th century women have already been recognized as legally capable as men (in her country, Israel, with the Constitution of 1948). According to Shalev, this is not enough: to pass the acid test for rationality, women must be able to treat their babies as commodities.[77]

Tabet (2014, 172 ff.) instead considers surrogate motherhood as the classical commodification of labor analysed by Marx: from servitude to contract. In the realm of procreation it might be an improvement, against a his-

---

[75] See in Teman (2010, 76) how much the Israeli surrogates apply rationality to detach themselves from any feeling towards the "contract child" in their womb. Three lustra later, Shalev must be really proud of them.

[76] But the contract itself can be seen as distorting rationality: "A surrogate contract is inherently manipulative, since the very form of the contract invokes commercial norms which, whether upheld by the law or by social custom only, imply that the mother should feel guilty and irresponsible for loving her own child" (Anderson 1990, 89).

[77] Shalev nevertheless presents herself as a feminist, in the wake of the disparaging opinion of pregnancy expressed by de Beauvoir and Firestone.

torical backdrop in which women's capacities to generate have been appropriated by the collective of men in slavery-like conditions. Violence was and is customarily applied to break women's resistance and use their sexual functions, reducing them to passive objects to be exploited according to men's necessities.

To get a price on reproductive services—as it has been in many places and times for sexual services—could enhance women's position in society. But while this is doubtful for developed countries, as women did regain power over procreative decisions (certainly not absolutely, but in relative terms), ethnographic work has shown that in fact this might be the case in India: "While some of these women are coerced into surrogacy by their families, many others are negotiating with their families to gain control over their own bodies and their fertility in order to participate in this process" (Pande 2014, 5). The "Eastern" and "Western" points of view—to hint at stereotypes—do not show the same position of women in the social hierarchy: class, as configured by stratification at the world-systemic level (not at the national one) must be taken into account.

The contract versus the agreement

The assault on *mater semper certa est*, and on the birth mother's final say on her relationship with the newborn, is well under way. Today these legal principles have ceased to be universal. Commodification of parental relationships is the direction of the present movement, especially since the development of ART. But only in a few places has the law already arrived where complete freedom of contract reigns over what was once considered a "parent's status," threatening the breach of the surrogacy contract with monetary sanctions or specific performance orders—though the examples presented, especially the Chinese case in a prohibitionist context, do prove that to perform this injustice states do not even need to validate the surrogacy contract: an alleged "best interest of the child" is enough.[78] California, Greece and Tabasco (Mexico) are the only states that enforce surrogacy contracts even for a child not genetically related to the intended parents, establishing joint

---

[78] The cases might be very different from each other due to different states' laws in the US, but a synthesized datum is that all the 12 litigations in the '80s and early '90s were sentenced in favor of the commissioning parents: 11 couples and one father (Spitz 1996, 70, quoting the Center for Surrogate Parenting Newsletter, Spring 1993).

parenthood only by intention—that is, by the purchase of other people's genetic material. In India *de facto* "anything goes," though this is not admitted by the law.

But let us follow the chronological order of the approval of surrogacy contracts. California was the first to validate them in 1993, and in 2013 both the California Uniform Parentage Act and a law on surrogacy[79] were approved, listing giving birth, genetic consanguinity, intention, and being married to the genetic father or mother as valid proof of parenthood. Thus motherhood can be established by a piece of paper, and parenthood attributed even to genetically unrelated persons outside the adoption process. The statute also contains the possibility for a child to have more than two parents, if it is in its best interest (as judged by the courts).[80]

In 1996 Israel approved the Embryo Carrying Agreement Act, and established a Committee to evaluate surrogacy agreements. Petitioners must be a heterosexual couple resident in Israel and diagnosed with infertility, with a fertile intended father.[81] The surrogate mother must be unmarried and will receive compensation approved by the Committee. The parties are all evaluated by a psychologist and a social worker. Termination of pregnancy is limited to medical reasons. When the child is born:

> the intended parents receive the child temporarily in the presence of a governmental welfare agent, but the agent is the guardian of the child until a court decides otherwise. The intended parents must initiate proceedings for a decree called a Parenthood Order within seven days of the birth, otherwise the welfare agent will initiate such a procedure. A decree is granted unless the child's best interests demand otherwise, and so far no case in Israel has so demanded, thus the court's role largely concerns approving the parties' arrangement and granting the decrees. A surrogate's wish to keep the child is not in itself a reason not to grant a decree. However, if a social worker's review demonstrates that there has been a change in circumstances which justifies the surrogate's change of heart, and that it would not harm the best interest of the child, the court may grant her request. The Committee recommends that circumstances such as would justify a change

---

[79] "An action to establish the parent-child relationship between the intended parent or parents and the child as to a child conceived pursuant to an assisted reproduction agreement for gestational carriers may be filed before the child's birth, or the county where medical procedures pursuant to the agreement are to be performed. A copy of the assisted reproduction agreement for gestational carriers shall be lodged in the court action filed for the purpose of establishing the parent-child relationship" (AB-1217 Surrogacy agreements).

[80] There have been some cases in Canadian courts, too, see "Who is a Parent? Not a Simple Question!" by Stephanie Laskoski (http://www.lawnow.org/parent-simple-question/ accessed 15.3.2015).

[81] In her review of Teman's work (2010), Barbara Katz Rothman (2012) corrects the Israeli terminology of "intended mother" in "purchasing mother."

be stated in the original surrogacy agreement. So far no petition has ever been filed by a surrogate requesting to keep the child. (Shakargy 2013, 234)

The legal expert Sharon Shakargy so comments:"Clearly, the governing principle is the best interests of the child, but so is upholding the agreement. The legitimate interests of the surrogate are considered only when there has been an unforeseeable change of circumstances, and when the best interests of the child would not be compromised" (Shakargy 2013, 236). Clearly, the best interest of the child is not to be separated from its birth mother and from her nourishment, but this is muddled by another hocus pocus, as Shakargy declares the developing child well aware of its genes—and only of them: "The Act further requires that the surrogate must not be the egg donor, based on the best interest of the child in having a minimal connection to the woman who 'gave him (or her) up'" (Shakargy 2013, 237). The surrogate must be single because of the application of religious law in personal matters: in Judaism if a married woman begets a child but not with her husband, this child is a *mamzer*, which is a religious status (meaning "bastard"). A *mamzer* has diminished legal capacities, for example he or she and their descendants can marry only other *mamzerim*. In necessity, this rule of singlehood can and has been glossed over:

> Indeed, in 2006 there was one such case, in which the intended parents found a married woman who was willing to carry their child altruistically when they were unable to find any other surrogate due to financial difficulties. After long deliberations that involved the Chief Rabbi of Israel and the Knesset (Israeli Parliament), the procedure was approved. Since then, and due to the great difficulty in finding suitable surrogates, a few married surrogates have been approved. (Shakargy 2013, 236)

Contracts—and pro-natalism—are trumping religious dogmas even in Israel, now on its way to become a fully confessional state.

The Tabasco state of Mexico admitted contracts for gestational surrogacy in its civil code of 1997, not requiring genetic parenthood and assimilating traditional surrogacy to adoption, instead:

> In the case of children born as a result of the participation of a substitute gestational mother, the maternity of the intending mother who presents it will be presumed since that fact implies its acceptance. In cases involving a surrogate mother, the same requirement must be complied with as in full adoption. (Art. 92, § 4 Tabasco Civil Code, quoted by Lamm 2013a, 256–7)

Eleonora Lamm notes that the exact procedures are not specified, though the document to be presented should be a contract signed before a public notary.

In 2005 parenthood by genetics plus intention superseded *mater semper certa est* also in Illinois. The Gestational Surrogacy Act came into force "to provide legal certainty about parenthood for children born through gestational surrogacy arrangements" (European Parliament 2013, 49). This is a staple argument in favor of binding contracts: the uncertainty that must be cleared is in reality the true will of the birth mother. Broad control on pregnancy is accorded to the intended parents, as the surrogate must obey all clauses of the contract. As in California, the surrogate mother can be paid whatever amount without legal caps, and she will never be recognized as the mother at child's birth. These processes of commodification, in my view, are to be interpreted in relation to hegemony in the world-economy and not to Anglo-Saxon legal culture: what is important is not the cultural climate but the expansion of the monetary sphere, as the world-systems perspective shows (e.g. Wallerstein 2004).

But money is not even an issue in establishing binding contracts, as altruistic gestational surrogacy is configured with the same unappealable obligations in both South Africa and Greece. Greece legalized surrogacy contracts in 2002,[82] probably in its eagerness to "modernize" the country at the turn of the century, a period of booming economic investment for the Olympic Games and extravagant state expenditure for their preparation and for the purchase of weapons made in Germany and France, creating a public debt that ultimately ruined the Greek people.[83]

---

[82] The Greek provisions only partially satisfy Aristides N. Hatzis (2009, 2010), who studied at the University of Chicago Law School and did his PhD under the supervision of Richard A. Posner (see his proposals to establish markets in babies: Landes and Posner 1978, Posner 1987 and 1989). Hatzis deplores the cap on compensation to the breeder (my translation) and the restriction of surrogacy to residents in Greece. In times of global markets, this makes little sense indeed.

[83] In Greece surrogacy occurs both in legal and illegal ways: "In November 2006, after my lecture at the Panhellenic Conference of Midwives many of them approached me to inform me that they have witnessed not only commercial but also unreported surrogacies in their hospitals (both private and public). According to them it is quite easy to have an unreported surrogacy: the surrogate gives birth to the child in the hospital and the certificate is issued under the name of the commissioning mother posing as the biological mother. Some of them even insisted that unreported surrogacies are more frequent than the reported ones" (Hatzis 2010, 11, n. 15). This corruption, I believe, would not have hap-

According to Rethimiotaki (2008) and Rokas (2013), the Greek parliament took the step of liberalizing ART and regulating surrogacy as a pronatalist measure in the context of a declining birth rate[84] (capitalism requires the multiplication of its workforce, see Danna 2014). The rules require domicile in Greece, so reproductive tourism is thought to be discouraged, despite the evident advertising of Greek clinics over the internet in many languages: the residence requirement can be interpreted by the judge as only a temporary residence.[85] A medical reason for the intended mother not to undergo pregnancy is required. Rokas made an analysis of 136 traced court decisions allowing surrogacy since it started, in the period 2002–2011 (but probably there are many more, both official and unofficial). He found that over the half of the registered agreements involved foreigners: in 54% of the cases the surrogates, designed as "the best friends" of the intended mothers, came from Eastern Europe, and in most of the cases their role as breeders must have been an extension of the domestic work that migrant women do, probably for the same family. In a quarter of the cases the surrogate was a

---

pened without the legitimation of contracts in 2002, which gave infertile people the idea of the feasibility of this option.

[84] The initiative is recounted in this way: "On November 22, 2000 the Minister of Justice, at the time Mihail Stathopoulos, a leading academic of Law at Athens Law School, and a man with a progressive mind, appointed a Committee to evaluate the effects of the RTs [reproductive technologies] and genetics to family law. The result of this project was the formation and the passing of the Law 3089/2002 on December 19, 2002" (European Parliament 2013, 279). The Parliament modified it prohibiting financial gains and forbidding traditional surrogacy. The Report to the European Parliament praises the law disguising its meaning with a mountain of lies: "First and foremost, it aims to protect the rights and interests of any resulting child [which to the contrary is not to be separated from its mother], and secondly the individuals' right to personal freedom and autonomy [but for the breeder's], and their right to procreate [which doubtfully exists for the infertile, and most certainly not at the expense of other persons]. Consequently, [the biggest lies follow] Laws 3089/2002 and 3305/2005 are in harmony with the national legislation in general, as well as the moral principles, rights and obligations incorporated into the Greek Constitution, while at the same time they are consistent with the European and international laws and inter-countries' agreements on Human Rights and on the protection of and respect for the children's welfare" (European Parliament 2013, 277-8). They are not: international conventions affirm the right to be brought up by one's family and, on the side of the mother, the protection of her family life.

[85] Controls that are only formal are not an obstacle to all kinds of arrangements: "A former client of mine, an American citizen, asked my opinion about having a child through surrogacy in Greece. When I informed him on the conditions and the prohibitions he was amazed. In his correspondence with a fertility clinic in Greece the issue of non residency never came up and the problem of the surrogate mother was not an issue. The fertility clinic even had a catalogue with possible candidates" (Hatzis 2010, 11, n. 16).

member of the family: mother, sister or sister-in-law of the woman petitioning.

As the agreement must be altruistic, no advertisement is permitted, and there is a cap on the sums that can be given:

> The woman who gestates and gives birth for another woman is compensated for all the expenses which are necessary for achieving pregnancy, the gestation and the parturition, provided that those are not covered by her social security fund. The amount that will be paid results from the receipts issued in conformity with tax law. Those expenses are recoverable only if the judicial permission necessary for surrogacy has been granted. [...] The woman who bears a child for another woman, is compensated for her absence from her work, which is necessary to achieve pregnancy, the gestation, the parturition and the puerperium. [...] If the gestating woman is unemployed, the amount of her compensation covers the fee which she, in accordance to her professional qualifications, would receive if she was working. In no case shall the compensation exceed the amount of 10,000 EUR. The compensation is due only if the judicial authorization required by law is granted. (Ministerial Decision no. 36, art. 2 and 4 [OG B' 670/16.04.2009] quoted by Rokas 2013, 147, n. 11)

But Rokas writes that it seems common that, under the table, bigger sums change hands.

As in Israel, no conflict has been brought to litigation yet: "No case has been reported where a surrogate mother has been opposed to the intended parents on any point" (Rokas 2013, 147). This is commented upon as a sign of the well functioning of the regulation: "The almost complete nonexistence [but why then "no case" just above?] of judicial controversies in relation to surrogacy in past years constitutes an indication that this new institution is functioning well in the country" (Rokas 2013, 165), without giving so much as a second thought to the power dynamics between migrant domestic workers and well-to-do Greek couples.

The surrogacy contracts must be approved by a tribunal before the woman gets pregnant, but tribunals have validated contracts even after. The judge just looks at the written agreement, from which its altruistic character must result (an incisive measure!), as well as the domicile in Greece. A heterosexual couple or a single woman can be the actors, with medical reasons not to be able to give birth. The prospective surrogate must be evaluated also psychologically, but she must not submit herself to any condition other than giving up the baby, retrieving her full autonomy on the rest, for example in respect to abortion (it is fortunate that the contract cannot go against Greek laws!).

The article of the Civil Code establishing this exception to *mater semper certa est* is Article 1464, as modified by the Law 3089/2002 on Medically Assisted Human Reproduction:

> In case that the child is born after medically assisted reproduction of a surrogate mother, under the conditions of article 1458,[86] it is presumed that mother is the one who has obtained the Court permission.
> This presumption can be reversed by a legal action contesting the maternity, within six months from the birth of the child. The maternity can be contested by legal action either by the presumed mother or by the surrogate mother, provided that evidence is produced that the child is issued biologically by the latter [το τέκνο κατάγεται βιολογικά από την τελευταία]. The contesting must be proceeded with by the woman entitled to do so personally or by her specially authorized attorney or by the Court permission by her lawful representative.
> Following the irrevocable Court decision that admits the legal action, mother of the child is considered to be the surrogate mother [literally "the woman who has gestated it:" τη γυναίκα που το κυοφόρησε] with retroactive effect as from the fact of its birth.[87]

The commentators I read are unanimous that "biologically issued" here means "from one's egg," that is: a maternity suit could be admitted only in cases of a conception by "error" with the birth mother's egg. But this has not been proved in a tribunal yet—and can never be proved with biology itself (see Rethimiotaki 2015). But apart from the very much presumed different treatment of gestational and traditional surrogacy in Greek law, another paradox is the concept of "altruistic surrogacy contract" itself. How can surrogacy be altruistic if it is ultimately coerced?

The fifth state to give the green light to contracts depriving birth mothers of their rights already *in utero* was Ukraine, according to the spirit of perfect gender equality of Article 123 of The Ukrainian Family Code, as amended December 22, 2006 (No. 524-V):

---

[86] *Article 1458*. The transfer of fertilized ova to another woman and pregnancy by her is allowed by a court authorization issued before the transfer, given that there is a written and, without any financial benefit, agreement between the involved parties, meaning the persons wishing to have a child and the surrogate mother and in case that the latter is married of her spouse, as well. The court authorization is issued following an application of the woman who wants to have a child, provided that evidence is adduced not only in regard with the fact that she is medically unable to conceive but also with the fact that the surrogate mother is in good health condition and able to conceive" (http://policy.mofcom.gov.cn/english/flaw!fetch.action?libcode=flaw&id=28fb9603-75e9-4691-a960-36b0d9a2c624&classcode=330 accessed 26.12.2014).

[87] http://policy.mofcom.gov.cn/english/flaw!fetch.action?libcode=flaw&id=28fb9603-75e9-4691-a960-36b0d9a2c624&classcode=330 accessed 26.12.2014.

Article 123. Establishing Maternal and Paternal Affiliation in Case of Medically Assisted Procreation and Ovum Implantation
1. If the wife is fertilized by artificial procreation techniques upon written consent of her husband, the latter is registered as the father of the child born by his wife.
2. If an ovum [original: embryo] conceived by the spouses is implanted to another woman, the spouses shall be the parents of the child.
3. Whenever an ovum conceived by the husband with another woman is implanted to his wife, the child is cnsidered to be affiliated to the spouses.[88]

Consent to the agreement by the surrogate mother must be notarized according to the Rules of Civil Registration, and no case of litigation is known (Druzenko 2013, 358).

South Africa was the sixth state in 2010 to transform the agreement into a legally valid contract after a court's stamp of approval. There are two kinds of coercion that force the consent of the surrogate: specific performance enforcement, that is the state helping the intended parents to take the child without the consent of the birth mother, and economic coercion: the surrogate mother being forced to give back the money received and even compensate for "damages." In South Africa they apply, respectively, in the two situations of gestational and traditional surrogacy:

> A surrogate mother who is also a genetic parent of the child concerned may at any time prior to the lapse of a period of sixty days after the birth of the child, terminate the surrogate motherhood agreement by filing written notice with the court (Children's Act 2005, s. 298 § 1, rules implemented in 2010)

But this change of heart is not free:

> The surrogate mother incurs no liability to the commissioning parents for exercising her right of termination in terms of this section, except for compensation for any payments made by the commissioning parents in terms of section 301 [regulating the reimbursement]. (Children's Act 2005, s. 298 § 3)

It is obvious that women willing to become a surrogate in their vast majority have already spent the sums received for their necessities of sheer survival, as it is also meant by laws capping the "reimbursement." On the contrary, in situations of private or agency adoption in the US, if the would-be adopters paid for the expenses of the birth mother, she is not under any obligation to

---

[88] As translated by www.familylaw.com (original: http://zakon4.rada.gov.ua/laws/show/2947-14 both accessed 20.1.2015). This and the other typos in the quoted sentences are identical in the original.

give the sum back: payment for her needs is not conditional on her surrendering her child, but it is considered a liberal act from the rich.

Other conditions in South Africa are also similar to the Greek rules: only "altruistic" surrogacy is admitted, but here the judge can dispose inspections to make sure that the agreement reports the true situation. Curious indeed, the birth mother is the only one who cannot act with economic aims, while the intended parents use their money to force her, and doctors, clinics and lawyers take their good share of the deal as professional legal and medical services are legally entitled to "reasonable compensation" (Children's Act s. 301 § 3).

Same-sex couples and also single men can apply for surrogacy because of the anti-discrimination constitutional provision about marital status and sexual orientation, provided the petitioners have a genetic link with the child. South Africa prohibits agencies and publicity, requests psychological evaluation of the surrogate, allows only for reimbursement and compels the commissioning parents to stipulate a life insurance for the surrogate:

> No promise or agreement for the payment of any compensation to a surrogate mother or any other person in connection with a surrogate motherhood agreement or the execution of such an agreement is enforceable, except a claim for-
> (a) compensation for expenses that relate directly to the artificial fertilisation and pregnancy of the surrogate mother, the birth of the child and the confirmation of the surrogate motherhood agreement;
> (b) loss of earnings suffered by the surrogate mother as a result of the surrogate motherhood agreement; or
> (c) insurance to cover the surrogate mother for anything that may lead to death or disability brought about by the pregnancy. (s. 301 § 2)

Can the surrogacy agreement—in particular, but not only, when deemed "altruistic"—be a proper juridical transaction? According to Ines Corti, the answer is "no:"

> This configuration results problematic. It is not possible indeed to hypothesize that the woman who put her body at the disposal of other persons with their own reproductive ends should have the obligation to have the embryo implanted in her, or to give the ovum for fecundation (in the case she is also the genetic mother), not to interrupt her pregnancy (or to interrupt it in case certain events occur, for example the acknowledgement of an handicap in the fetus), to submit herself to medical care during pregnancy, to maintain a certain conduct during this period, and in the end to give up the baby. These obligations would affect the freedom of the woman, limiting some of her fundamental rights. (Corti 2000, 180)

The contract, instead, entitling the intended parents not only from a legal but also from a cultural point of view to a gestational service or product (according to the different interpretations) dehumanizes maternity. A verdict of the Tribunale di Rimini in 1995 clearly showed *a contrario* that motherhood by intention is impossible to achieve without an objectifying view of the woman who undergoes pregnancy. This Tribunal denied the inscription of an "intended father" on the birth certificate of a child conceived with "donor sperm" by his wife, ordering him to make a request for adoption to the Court for minors. In the spirit of gender equality, the Tribunal speculated:

> In the same manner through the "renting of the womb," biological motherhood must be attributed to the "donor" of the fertilized egg, notwithstanding that pregnancy is conducted to term by another woman, who essentially has the function of "incubator." (Tribunale di Rimini 1996, 581)

This interpretation, according to the tribunal, is the only one that would respect the obligation not to alter the civil status of the infant and its *real* relationships of procreation and lineage. "Real" (the inverted commas were used by the Tribunal—a sign of feeling shameful?) is an attribute applied to genetic origin, leaping the stage of pregnancy. As said, since pregnancy is not a male experience, this might be the reason why tribunals do not acknowledge its reality—as in this other verdict by a New Zealand court:

> A New Zealand Family Court judge observed in 2008 that the presumption that the mother of the child is the person who gives birth to that child, even in the face of that woman having no genetic relationship to the child, means that in surrogacy situations in New Zealand, "the true reality of the situation, that is, the genetic reality, is not recognized by law." (*In the matter of C [Adoption]* [2008] New Zealand Family Law Reports 141, para [31] per Judge Walsh, quoted by Ahmed 2013, 302)

When men, or tribunals representing male power, decide upon the meaning of pregnancy, they trivialize it.

Martha Field (1988, 78) affirms that "the law should make the contract performable or not at the option of the mother," as she has to waive what in the US is a constitutional right to her progeny. Some commentators argue that what is being sold in surrogacy are "the reproductive services" of a woman, but this is just a lawyer's rhetorical trick: when a mechanic repairs a car selling his or her mechanical services, or when a hairdresser cuts hair, the car and the hair are already there—but a baby is neither repaired nor coiffed: what happens in contract surrogacy is what happens when one instead buys a new car or a new wig. Services are famously distinguished from goods as "something that cannot fall on your feet" and I would say that a newborn will fall, and—more than hurt you—be hurt in consequence.[89]

For Mary Lyndon Shanley, gestational work cannot be assimilated to a job to be performed for others:

> Human gestation is distinguished from other kinds of productive work, however, by the ways in which it involves both a woman's physical and psychological being and by the difference between the human being that results from a pregnancy and other kinds of products. (Shanley 1993, 626)

Elizabeth Anderson writes against this kind of commodification: "Treating women's labor as just another kind of commercial production process violates the precious emotional ties which the mother may rightly and properly establish with her 'product,' the child." When a woman is required "to repress whatever parental love she feels for the child, these [economic] norms convert women's labor into a form of alienated labor" (Anderson 1990). We will see in next chapter how true this is.

The social view of the birth mother affirmed by the legal validity and enforceability of the surrogacy contract is that she is a breeder for someone else: for the upper class (or even the middle class, especially in international surrogacy performed in poor countries). In this vision, the birth mother is simply considered as a vessel for somebody else's genome, a vehicle for a fetus, as Janice Raymond wrote. For Margaret Radin, in surrogacy women are considered fungible in carrying on the male genetic line (Radin 1996, 142), and Scott Rae (1994, 63) writes: "Thus the service that surrogates perform, particularly if the surrogate contributes the egg, involves a misconception about her role as the child's mother, and treats the woman as a reproductive vessel, carrying the precious genetic cargo of the man." Martha Field (1988, 50) finds that among the motives of contracting fathers the desire to reproduce oneself might not be the healthiest in order to found a family: if the father is so focused upon half the genes of his offspring, what if the child turns out to chiefly resemble its mother, instead? Some legal experts

---

[89] Also Scott Rae writes against the interpretation in terms of "service": "The child that is born out of a physician's expertise has no relationship to the physician, and the physician has no claim to any parental rights. Likewise, the adoption attorney is being paid so that a couple can obtain a child. But it is not the attorney's child that they are obtaining. This is not the case with surrogacy. The child for which the money is being paid is the legal child of the surrogate, and the fee is paying for much more than just gestational services" (Rae 1994, 52).

argue instead for contracts analogous to all other working relationships: John Dwight Ingram (1993) titles his article "Surrogate gestator: a new and honorable profession." To the contrary, Alayna Ohs arrives at the conclusion that surrogacy can only be conceived of as labor if legislation allows for slavery:

> Regardless of the possible issues of commodification, this fails to account for the reality that gestation is not like other forms of labour. Unlike an at-will employment situation, for example, requiring specific performance of a surrogacy agreement would violate the Constitution because it would result in involuntary servitude—by forcing a woman to carry a child to term, the court would be forcing a performance of her 'services.' Though courts have generally rejected this argument, it is disingenuous for them to have it both ways—to characterize a surrogacy contract as a contract for "services," as the Johnson court did, and then to deny that forcing a woman to complete a pregnancy is coerced labour. (Ohs 2002, 360–361)

Many users and advocates of surrogacy identify it with the contract that permits the automatic inscription on the birth certificate itself of the name of the commissioning parent. But this is not the only way to establish such an agreement. In the first chapter I have described the possibility of private understandings—and sometimes these are supported and regulated with strong requirements, guaranteeing in exchange a fast adoption track: in the Netherlands the Child Protection Board oversees gestational surrogacy, allowing for a reflection period for the birth mother before she definitively has to give the baby to the intended parents. As far as traditional surrogacy is concerned, all children's placement in the Netherlands must be supervised by this governmental agency.

Regulations and slippery slopes

In all other countries of the world but for the six where the surrogacy contract is legally valid, agreements are not protected by law as contracts. They are fulfilled only after the final consent of the birth mother to relinquish the child and her parental duties and responsibilities towards it. The situation in the EU countries shows the spectrum of possibilities: in some legislations the intended parents' names appear on a new birth certificate, cancelling the legal traces of the birth mother, as in anonymous delivery, while other legislators reacted to the novelty of IVF and embryo transfer by nipping them in the bud with a prohibition (see the table 4 in European Parliament 2013, 15–16). In Germany the law of 1990 not only forbids ovum donations, but provides penal sanctions to the doctors performing it. The aim is explicitly to preserve the connection between ovum, pregnancy and social motherhood. France and Italy are also prohibitionist in regard not only to surrogacy but to other IVF procedures. Other countries with a general prohibition of surrogacy are Malta, Portugal, and Spain. Egg commerce is prohibited in Austria. Only commercial surrogacy is prohibited in Belgium, Denmark, Greece (where "altruistic" surrogacy is performed by migrants), Hungary, Ireland, Latvia, and the UK; Finland and Sweden prohibit the use of all ART in relation to surrogacy.

In Belgium, Denmark, the Netherlands, and Sweden adoption is required to transfer parenthood, while in the UK Parental Orders transfer parenthood in an easier way than the adoption procedure. In Bulgaria and Sweden a general prohibition is affirmed, but legislative proposals to accept and regulate some forms of surrogacy are currently being discussed, while in 2010 they were rejected in France and withdrawn in Rumania.

The few countries which regulate surrogacy apply different models to its agreements which can be distinguished by a few variables. There is in fact no international consensus on how to deal with this issue, and regulations basically differ in the following ways, with the first alternative seemingly the most common:

1. only gestational surrogacy is regulated / also traditional surrogacy is;
2. the intended parents must have a genetic link with the child / they can buy all genetic material;
3. there must be a medical need (the intended mother is declared by a doctor unable to bring a pregnancy to term) / the sole will to outsource the pregnancy suffices;
4. negotiated compensation, including foregone gains, is allowed / only a reimbursement of expenses can be approved;
5. the intended parent(s) can only be heterosexual couples (sometimes only married couples) / also same-sex couples / also single women / also single men (generally none of them must be previously convicted of crimes);
6. they must be domiciled in the country / resident / have a medical visa / do not need any of these requirements;

7. the surrogate could be asked to meet certain requirements in terms of age, marital status, criminal record, previous pregnancies, no desire for other children, psychological health, and of course physical fitness.

Another variable concerns the possibility of penal punishment for doctors who perform ART in unapproved (or in all) surrogacy contexts for agencies to broker surrogacy agreements, and for advertisements to be published: it is generally considered ethical to let surrogacy agreements be reached only between the intended parents and the woman willing to help, without being pushed by third parties (agencies, clinics, lawyers).

And, of course, there is the variable that we have already described: is the birth mother punished if she takes back her consent after signing the contract and becoming pregnant, or can she have a reflection period after birth? Among the states positively regulating surrogacy, the majority allows for a "change of heart" period: only those described in the previous paragraph do not. The problem is that very often this only happens on paper. Even the states where "reproductive tourism" is directed, like India and Russia, have provisions that allow for the birth mother to keep the baby, but it is not very likely that these women really have a choice. The Russian civil code allows for exceptions to *mater semper certa est* only with the post-partum consent of the birth mother,[90] and there should be some possibility to deny it, as the clinics do not monitor the whole process (but agencies do, if the surrogacy arrangements have not been made independently, without mediators).[91] But in India the clinics hold surrogate mothers in a very subordinate position. In 2012 India introduced the requirement to intended parents of having a medical visa: to access surrogacy legally they must be a heterosexual couple married at least for two years, and they "must" verify at their Embassy that the procedure will be approved—without presenting evidence of such an approval. To avoid completely the problem of babies being stopped at the border, India should have made the presentation of an official docu-

---

[90] Family Code of Russia, 1995, s. 51, para 4(2) "a married couple that has given its consent in written form to implantation of an embryo into another woman for the purpose of its gestation, can be registered as the child's parents only with the consent of this woman (surrogate mother)" (quoted by Khazova 2013, 313).

[91] Christina Weis, doing a PhD with participant observation of surrogacy in Russia, affirms that it is not practised only in big cities but throughout Russia. Surrogate mothers are mostly Russians, but also Ukrainians, Moldovans and Belarussians, who come to Russia for surrogacy (Weis 2014 and email correspondence on file with author).

ment from an embassy compulsory before the procedure starts. But this would go against its public policy of incentivizing medical tourism.

The Indian guidelines, in force since 2005,[92] regulate gestational surrogacy, defining it as "an arrangement in which a woman agrees to carry a pregnancy that is genetically unrelated to her and her husband, with the intention to carry it to term and hand over the child to the genetic parents for whom she is acting as a surrogate" (Ministry of Health 2005, § 1.2.33). Abortion remains a right of the surrogate. The intended parents have a preferential right to adopt the child after the six week's delay mandated for the expression of maternal consent with a notarized agreement. The woman carrying the child remains its birth mother but—again—intended parents can claim custody in the best interest of the child.

In Brazil surrogacy is regulated by the Federal Medical Board (Conselho Federal de Medicina) that establishes:

> *VII - Surrogacy (temporary doration of uterus):*
> The Clinics and centres for reproductive services can use assisted reproductive techniques to create a situation identified as surrogacy, as long as there is a medical problem that prevents the intended mother from having a baby [but not from donating eggs].
> 1) The surrogate mothers must belong to the same family as the intended mother, up to the second degree. All other cases are subject to authorization of the Regional Medical Board.
> 2) The surrogate situation cannot be commercial. (de Araujo 2013, 85)

An article specifies that the expenses of the pregnant woman can be paid: food, clothes and education (Padilha Fernandes 2014).

Also in Australia commercial surrogacy is a criminal offence, and there must be a medical necessity for altruistic surrogacy, which must be gestational and is forbidden to singles. It must be done with counseling for all parties, unenforceable contracts, and acquisition of parentage through adoption with a "parentage order." Only reasonable expenses related to pregnancy can be reimbursed, where "reasonable" stands for incurred and verifiable. But in four states this also means "recovery of lost income" (Keyes 2013,

---

[92] Usha Rengachary Smerdon writes: "Critics challenge the Guidelines on numerous grounds. Commentators note that the Guidelines reinforce social prejudices toward infertility without stressing the need for the prevention of infertility. Informed consent is dealt with in a vague and cursory manner and is not even made mandatory under the Guidelines," as the birth certificate shall be in the name of the intended parents (Smerdon 2008, 41).

33). Tasmania completely forbids the agreements with the Surrogacy Contracts act 1993.

New Zealand does not make any difference between traditional and gestational surrogacy. They are both considered "an arrangement under which a woman agrees to become pregnant for the purpose of surrendering custody of a child born as a result of her pregnancy." The agreement is unenforceable in either case: "A surrogacy agreement is not itself illegal, but is not enforceable by or against any person." Not all payments are prohibited, only "valuable consideration," and organizing commercial surrogacy is a criminal offence:

> Every person commits an offence who gives or receives, or agrees to give or receive, valuable consideration for his or her participation, or for any other person's participation, or for arranging any other person's participation, in a surrogacy arrangement.[93]

In Canada only altruistic surrogacy is allowed, and loss of income is included in the reimbursable expenses.

To conclude this quick view of surrogacy regulation around the world, the US—as usual—is a true patchwork of provisions. We have seen the (de)regulation in California and in Illinois. Also in Florida, Nevada, New Hampshire, and Virginia the contracts are valid, provided that a court approves them: there must be a medical reason to enter them, and the parties must be psychologically evaluated. Only in Virginia is the law on surrogacy modelled after the regulation of adoption, with a guardian ad litem nominated by the court to represent the future child and a home visit to the intended parents—only married couples—by the social services. A second group of states only allows for altruistic surrogacy, that is, noncompensated agreements: Kentucky, Louisiana, Maryland, Nebraska, and Washington.[94] In Alabama, Iowa, and West Virginia contracts are admitted, and they are explicit-

---

[93] Section 5, section 14, and section 14(3) of the Human Assisted Reproductive Technology Act 2004 (all quoted in Achmad 2013, 297-8).

[94] It looks like nobody controls, though: "I was a gs, so the baby wasn't mine. from what i understand, hubby and I automatically are considered the "parents"for the bc. My IF had KY attorneys go to court with an affadavit stating that i wasn't the mother, I signed all my rights away, and named him as the father. Later, they are using MA lawyers to do a stepparent adoption for my IM, since she and I are both not the "mother". It was an egg donor. Oh, and this was all a FET too. [...] The philosophy is that my surrobabe was mine, and what I wanted to do with her when I left was up to me. They said they're just trying to cover their butts in case something happened. (I guess like if I changed my mind)" (posted on http://www.surromomsonline.com/support/showthread.php?156123-Surrogacy-laws-in-Kentucky11.11.2009, accessed 15.2.2015).

ly exempted from the provisions forbidding the sale of babies. Surrogacy contracts are void in the following states: Arizona, the District of Columbia, Indiana, Michigan, New York, North Dakota, and Utah. In all other states, about half, the Baby M case is considered a precedent:

> In states that have not addressed the subject by statute, issues regarding the lawfulness and enforceability of surrogacy contracts are resolved by courts in a manner similar to how the *Baby M* case was resolved, that is, by determining the best interests of the child and weighing any competing public policy concerns.[95]

But in some of the other states Pre-Birth Orders are applied: "Also known as the Petition for Declaratory Judgment, the Pre-Birth Order is just what it sounds like—an order established prior to the birth of the child that details the parent names to be listed on the birth certificate and more" (Alexander 2006, 73). The states applying it, according to Alexander, were Arkansas, California, Colorado; Connecticut, Georgia, Florida, Illinois, Kansas, Maryland, Massachusetts, Minnesota, Montana, Nevada, North Carolina, Ohio, Oklahoma, Oregon (judged rare), Pennsylvania, Texas and Utah. All the legal frameworks regulating surrogacy deny that surrogate mothers are working: they are not compensated but reimbursed, and they never pay taxes on the cash they receive.

Let us now go back to some of the points listed above to show that in crucial questions regulations display dangerous slippery slopes. In general I am not particularly sympathetic with the "slippery slope" argument, as it is often based on speculation and it is used to create unjustified fears. But in matters of surrogacy it is based on some facts. "Regulation" itself is asked for by the powerful advocates of surrogacy, speaking for the dominant capitalist class, who want all the legal guarantees to be able to buy life itself. "Regulation" then just means legalization, as Herbert Krimmel pointed out:

> In other words, it is precisely because they do fear that surrogacy can be stopped that they are trying so hard to get legislation passed "regulating" (read: permitting) the practice. As Clausewitz said about war, victory is achieved when you destroy your enemy's will to resist. If legislators can be convinced that laws against surrogacy are futile, then the proponents of surrogacy will indeed have won. (Krimmel 1992, 3)

---

[95] Law Library - American Law and Legal Information 2014: in Re Baby M - Further Readings - Child, Court, Contract, and Whitehead - JRank Articles http://law.jrank.org/pages/4604/Baby-M-in-Re.html#ixzz3Mvs3vGGB accessed 22.12.2014.

Krimmel also argues that the section 273 of the California Penal Code, prohibiting brokering and baby-selling in adoption should be logically applied to surrogacy. This is the provision:

> (a) It is a misdemeanor for any person or agency to offer to pay money or anything of value, or to pay money or anything of value, to a parent for the placement for adoption, for the consent to an adoption, or for cooperation in the completion of an adoption of his or her child. (b) This section does not make it unlawful to pay the maternity connected medical or hospital and necessary living expenses of the mother preceding and during confinement as an act of charity, as long as the payment is not contingent upon placement of the child for adoption, consent to the adoption, or cooperation in the completion of the adoption.[96]

Plus in some states no living expenses can be paid, only medical costs. Krimmel believes that "Commercial surrogacy falls within the clear language of statutes such as this one; moreover, applying statutes such as this to surrogacy would be perfectly consistent with their central purpose: to prevent children from being treated as items of commerce" (Krimmel 1992, 4–5).

Legal experts advocating for commercial surrogacy have staple arguments: a typical one is the fear of a black market where worse things would happen than legally expropriating women of their offspring, e.g. "the lack of a legal regulation 'forces' the couple or person desirous of having a child to resort to the black market, and it expands the possible abuses and injustices" (Lamm 2013a, 11). This is easier said than done, as a "black market baby," must at some point be legalized—at least in countries with rule of law, from where most of the intended parents come from. A second argument used is "the uncertainty of status,"[97] that is legal jargon for the impossibility of changing at will the official registration of a child's mother: "The system [proposed by Lamm] is similar to the one regulated under Greek law. It protects against legal uncertainties and change of mind of the surrogate" (Lamm 2013a, 14). Here the writer (just an example among many) implies that the "change of mind" is something that the birth mother is not entitled to have: she must be coerced by a contract that automatically mandates the separa-

---

[96] Quoted by Krimmel (1992, 4-5) and still valid, see http://www.thestork.com/expense.html accessed 21.1.2015. See also the legal dispute in Michigan about the application to surrogacy of a similar provision (Parker 1982).

[97] It is also used to refer to the period when the child is raised by the intended parents but the parental responsibility lies (also) with the surrogate mother, during the reflection period. Emily Jackson (2006, 65) claims that "This sort of uncertainty, even if relatively short-lived, is clearly not in the best interest of the child," without providing any concrete case where this has resulted detrimental to it.

tion. A third argument is the injustice done when genetic intended mothers have to go through an adoption process to have a legal tie to the baby while their husbands did not. The law needed to cancel one mother to pretend that nothing had changed after IVF, and in order to create a market in babies, the birth mother was the one to go. Therefore the law can simply reinstate her, modifying the obsolete legal concept of parenthood, liberating it from what has become a lie: that the biological parents can only be two. But, as argued, rights that should be attached to the genetic contribution cannot be more than a recognition of genetic origin, while the familial relationship of the newborn must be determined by its birth mother.

Many regulations end up with the same unacceptable forced separation of the birth mother from her child, primarily by means of the social dynamics that transform a "reimbursement" into a salary. Rarely can we walk out on a job, especially a low-paying one such as this (in rich countries), because if we accepted it in the first place, it means that we are not doing very well financially. And in the case of pregnancy as a job, to walk out also means to give back all the pay that was previously received! The slippery slope is firmly in place regarding the pretended noncommercial nature of surrogacy particularly where reimbursement of extravagant expenses is allowed for, e.g. "living expenses," "foregone gains," "education." In some countries, the possibility of consent in surrogacy depends on the motivation, as women wanting to get a market price are discouraged. But reimbursement of foregone gains is a salary by another name, and when women get paid to surrender the child, a market in babies is created and regulated. Advocates of surrogacy are right in finding this kind of regulation hypocritical.

Easily subject to a slippery slope is the requisite of infertility: the medical reasons for having somebody else carry a baby are progressively dismissed, and the sole will to procreate is left. This is accomplished by the application to the existing provisions of the principle of nondiscrimination between fertile and infertile, and between men and women by the tribunals, who stretch the law to cover everyone.[98] The medical need for surrogacy is

---

[98] To contrast this assimilation of fertile and infertile, Martha Field (1988, 47) notes: "In one sense, the state has a rule for all—that all can have children naturally but not for hire—and that rule is probably not vulnerable to attack under the equal protection clause. Even though the couple is hurt by that rule, it is not unreasonable for the state to distinguish between pregnancy achieved naturally and pregnancy for hire, if they are substantially different things."

an impossibility for the intended mother to carry a pregnancy to term, but this is difficult to pinpoint, as age itself makes conception and gestation difficult. And if we admit that somebody else can furnish the eggs when the woman is infertile because she is too old, why insist on having at least a genetic link by the intended parents? If both members of the couple are sterile, why should not ART come to their rescue? But is there a right to reproduce for anybody using ART, just because the possibility is there? Advocates of ART even want the possibility to access them through the public health service—but is it in the common interest of our society to create genetically unrelated babies for the infertile?

It is sometimes argued that the constitutional right to the development of one's personality entails the right to make use of the advances in ART. From this, a right to use surrogacy is derived, which is clearly foul play, as surrogacy is not a "technique" but the use of a woman's body. The Report to the European Parliament even takes for granted this presumed constitutional right to procreate for the infertile, mistakenly attributed to both South African and Greek Constitutions: "The facilitation of surrogacy is based on the constitutional recognition of a right to have a child: art. 5 para. 1 of the Greek Constitution; s.12 (2) (a) of the SA Constitution" (European Parliament 2013, 42, table 7). But in the articles referred to, no explicit right to reproduce can be found, much less a right to do it using somebody else:

> Greek Constitution: "*Article 5: 1.* All persons shall have the right to develop freely their personality and to participate in the social, economic and political life of the country, insofar as they do not infringe the rights of others or violate the Constitution and the good usages."

> South African Constitution: "*Section 12.2.* Everyone has the right to bodily and psychological integrity, which includes the right *a.* to make decisions concerning reproduction; *b.* to security in and control over their body."

It is particularly ironic that the referenced clause of the Constitution of South Africa is found in the section about "Freedom and the security of the person," guaranteeing one's control over her body—so if the Report's interpretations were true, the consequence would be self-contradictory. Still, it would not be the first time: the general principle of nondiscrimination and equality between the sexes applied to procreation generates (legal) monsters, as in the Constitution of the United Mexican States, that has been even hailed as a feminist one, as it gave constitutional rank to reproductive rights. But its neutral formulation makes the provision outright ridiculous: "every person has the right to decide in a free, mature and informed way, the number and spacing of their Children" (Article 4 as quoted and translated by Lamm 2013a, 255).[99] The article contradicts itself: if the "person" is a woman, then her reproductive rights are defended, but if the "person" is a man, men have acquired the right to dominate women's reproductive behavior. Eleonora Lamm continues unabated: "This implies the recognition of reproductive rights and reproductive freedom, which could include surrogacy." Or rather could not, as a man's right in this matter equals a woman's slavery. The contrast of interest between the sexes is—for once—evident and clearclut.

What has been argued for by jurists in respect to these and other similar constitutional articles is only that citizens should have the right to access all available technologies to circumvent their infertility, but a right to reproduce can never entail the use of another person's body: either in surrogacy or in gamete "donation." In fact, an international convention—not quite honored—even prohibits the commerce in gametes: "The human body and its parts shall not, as such, give rise to financial gain," recites the article on "Prohibition of financial gain" of the Convention for the Protection of Human Rights and Dignity of the Human Being with Regard to Biology and Medicine (Oviedo, 1997). Admittedly, gametes are peculiar parts, being detachable, but we have seen what the harm and the risks of egg retrieving operations are.

In Italy a right to procreation entailing the use of a surrogate's body was argued for by the Tribunal of Rome in 2000:

> It must be recognized as a fundamental right of the person the right to become parents and to evaluate and decide the choices in relation to the need to procreate, specifying that the parent status can find fulfillment in adoption but also in the transmission of one's own genes, and therefore, in particular cases, it must be decided in favor of the validity of the contract for the substitute maternity.[100]

These particular cases were never spelled out. On the contrary, this presumed right was recently turned down by the Constitutional Court with the

---

[99] Here's the original Spanish: "Art. 4, § 2—Toda persona tiene derecho a decidir de manera libre, responsable e informada sobre el número y el espaciamiento de sus hijos" (§ 1 is the affirmation of gender equality: "El varón y la mujer son iguales ante la ley. Esta protegerá la organización y el desarrollo de la familia").

[100] Tribunale civile di Roma, sez XI, 14 febbraio 2000, giudice C. Schettini *Contratto in genere. Contratto di sostituzione di maternità in determinati casi. Validità* http://www.diritto.it/sentenze/magistratord/roma14_02_2000.html accessed 20.12.2014.

verdict 162/2014, while taking down other parts of the prohibitionist ART law 40/2004.

If this admissibility of surrogacy for everybody can be seen as an anti-discriminatory move, and has probably been approved in this spirit, the result is rather a trumping of adoption laws. Given the shortage of babies to adopt and the interest of states to multiply their citizens (though this preoccupation is generally restricted to the "racially pure") the loosening of requisites and regulations in surrogacy is clearly a move by authorities to furnish babies to whomever wants them. This extension of women's procreative rights to men risked to happen in cases of surrogacy in Greece, where the entitlement of single infertile women but not of single infertile men to surrogacy had first been considered by the tribunals as being discriminatory.

The infertile single men's petitions were finally struck down in appeal (Athens Efeteio 3357/2010), because—infertile or not—men can never give birth to a child due to their anatomy (Rethimiotaki 2015).

Let us look in some detail at another concrete example of a long-standing regulation: in the UK private altruistic arrangements should not be mediated by anyone and can be recognized by court after birth, with a fast-track adoption ensuing. Publicity and third parties are forbidden. Can this very reasonable model of regulation turn out to be on a slippery slope, too? Compensation should not exceed "reasonable terms," but this is not the main interest of the juries: *post factum*, even market compensations have been approved (e.g. 27,000 GBP to a Ukrainian lady). And in 2008 the conditions for approval of the agreement have been relaxed. The new rules, implemented in 2010, did not request certification of medical problems anymore, nor being a heterosexual married couple (now only singles are excluded). Correspondingly, the number of surrogacy agreements rose. While during the period from 1995 to 2007, between 33 and 50 Parental Orders were granted each year, in 2008, 75 were granted; 79 in 2009, 83 in 2010, after cancellation of stricter rules the total in 2011 jumped to 149 Parental Orders (Crawshaw, Blyth E, van den Akker 2013). A chain reaction has started: in 2014 a survey found that the majority of Britons is now in favor of openly remunerating the surrogate mothers,[101] while in the past the maximum rate

---

[101] The questions were: "In general, do you approve or disapprove of people using gestational surrogacy to have children?" 59% of the sample answered approve, and 31% disapprove; "Do you think it should be legal or not legal to pay a surrogate?" with 54% for legalization

of approval of surrogacy (not specifically in Britain) was only 25% (Ciccarelli and Beckman 2005, 29). The press has not been particularly favorable to birth mothers, with titles like "Sorry, but I'm keeping your babies."[102] Increasingly sympathetic attitudes towards surrogacy were also testified to by researchers (van den Akker 2007), and there is no dearth of legal experts asking for contracts to be recognized (e.g. Horsey 2010). As we will see in chapter 4, in their subculture British surrogate mothers consider themselves workers.

Avoiding the slippery slopes, an agreement is surely free if it has two qualities: it is unconstrained and it is unpaid. The countries listed up to now fulfill the first criterion, but not the second: no approved regulation says that the agreement must be free in the sense of gratuitous. Only the Netherlands seems to be a place where marketization of babies has been reined in with a clear listing of reimbursed expenses, though the authorities are struggling against "surrogacy tourism," especially towards India, Ukraine, California and Greece. Third parties are criminalized, and gestational surrogacy is limited to people who can furnish both gametes, while traditional surrogacy is not regulated, but the Child Protection Board must approve all transfer of authority over children, and unlawful placement of a child is subject to penal sanction. The "treatment" of the couple with gestational surrogacy can occur with the contribution of a woman whom they must find themselves, following the ministerial guidelines and the *Richtlijn Hoog-technologisch draagmoederschap* (Guidelines on high-technology surrogacy) issued in 1999 by the Dutch Society for Obstetrics and Gynecology. Not only medical but also psychological support is offered to get an informed consent for the procedure from all parties involved. The transfer of only two embryos is allowed. The intended mother must not be older than 40, as egg quality declines with age, and viable embryos are increasingly difficult to obtain from older women. The clinics may also require residency or nationality.[103] And of course the agreement must be altruistic—with only the reimbursement of documented

---

of payment, and 26% against (*British public: legalise paid surrogacy* https://yougov.co.uk/news/2014/08/08/british-public-legalise-commercial-surrogacies/ accessed 28,2,2015).

[102] Jo Knowsley "Surrogate mother says 'Sorry, but I'm keeping your babies'," *Mail on Sunday*, 17.12. 2006 http://www.dailymail.co.uk/femail/article-423125/Surrogate-mother-says-Sorry-Im-keeping-babies.html accessed 2.2.2015.

[103] *Hoogtechnologisch draagmoederschap, Richtlijn Nederlandse Veerenigung voor Obstetrie en Gynaecologie*, n. 18, January 1999 (http://nvog-documenten.nl/uploaded/docs/richtlijnen_pdf/18_hoog_draagmoeder.pdf accessed 28.1.2015).

expenses related to pregnancy, e.g. maternity clothes. The Report to the European Parliament estimated as 7,500 EUR the cost of surrogacy in the Netherlands. But the Dutch are reviewing their position, and they might cave in to commodification: the argument goes that to avoid "surrogacy tourism" local rules should be relaxed, though this has never been a tenable argument for other ethical questions—quite the contrary for all prohibited psychoactive substances for example.

Other moves contrasting the marketization of babies are adopted even in countries that attract many foreign customers to their clinics. After legal disputes about babies blocked at the border, in the Balaz twins case waiting two years for a legal solution, India, as seen, has moved towards moral suasion in the visa process. There is debate in Ukraine about a new law complying with the Adoption Convention: to pay a surrogate mother more than her expenses would be prohibited, and access to the contracts will be restricted to residents in Ukraine (Druzenko 2013, 359 and 264). In February 2015 Thailand outlawed agencies, advertising and surrogacy for foreigners.[104]

But new countries are becoming the destination for those looking for surrogacy agreements. There are people simply dissatisfied with the official requirements: many intended parents find it easier and quicker to spend money travelling to get a baby to come home with, being officially (if wrongly) declared its parents. Going to a poor country, the cost of the surrogate is a bargain. Especially international lawyers[105] seem to be the incarnation of market forces wanting to turn procreation into a saleable service, pushing slyly for the recognition of whatever arrangement has resulted in a newborn who must be then carried across borders on behalf of the members of the privileged classes who have no qualms about buying themselves a baby (very often to be raised by their employees), covering it up with rhetoric that denies the purchase.

---

[104] "Thailand's parliament approves bill banning commercial surrogacy. Decision follows several surrogacy scandals this year including Australian couple who left behind baby with Down's syndrome," *The Guardian*, 28.11.2014 (http://www.theguardian.com/world/2014/nov/28/thailand-parliament-bill-ban-commercial-surrogacy-baby-gammy accessed 20.1.2015). "Thailand bans commercial surrogacy for foreigners," *BBC Asia News* 20.2.2015 (http://www.bbc.co.uk/news/world-asia-31546717 accessed 23.2.2015).

[105] One of them was amused to hear that I was working on a research on surrogate motherhood: "This theme is fun!" she commented. Then she described with admiration the large amount of money that was given to a certain group to elaborate their international law proposal on the funny theme.

All the laws and guidelines allowing for some form of even capped but vague "reimbursement" have established a market for babies, also because of the extreme degree of social inequality and poverty reigning in destitute countries.

Suspended babies

Legalization of surrogacy contracts, or at least of their cross-border effects[106] is promoted by many, observing that an effect of prohibition is to generate cross-border fluxes of people going to the "surrogacy-friendly" countries—though it is never mentioned that the flux does also come from countries with regulations, as the rules always exclude someone (fertile, gay, single, too old), while for some intended parents the process is never fast enough or sure enough because of the mother's reflection period.[107] Desperation due to infertility, or ignorance, or the need to spend less money, or the desire to save it, lead many couples to break their countries' laws by going abroad[108] and coming back with a baby and its false birth certificate that breaks the *mater semper certa* rule:

---

[106] Curiously, a legal scholar from the US proposes to resolve the question of transnational surrogacy with deference: "A simple solution [...] is for the countries-of-origin of the intended parents to give full force and effect to the US court orders and judgments establishing the parentage of the intended parents and terminating the parental rights of the surrogate (and her husband, if any). This would be done under the principle of international comity," which the author's note incredibly explains so: "not as a matter of obligation but of deference and respect" (Snyder 2013, 387).

[107] "Help and advice re: surrogacy in USA" 17/08/14, 19:20. Hello,We are probably at the end of our IVF journey and considering surrogacy and adoption.We are a little worried about surrogacy in the UK due to the time it may take to find a host and the legal issues of not being seen as the mother and father to the courts.I wonder if the USA would be quicker and offer better legal protection?" (http://www.fertilityfriends.co.uk/ accessed 13.12.2014).

[108] These conditions make people break the law also in their own country. What I find the most bizarre of all stories came under judgment of a Moscow court in 2011. A woman ordered nephews by the dozen to compensate for the loss of her son: "a 58-year-old woman, whose son had died from cancer, applied to the medical clinic for IVF with the use of the donor's oocytes and her deceased son's sperm, to be carried out with the subsequent transfer of embryos to a surrogate mother. To be confident in the success of her undertaking, the woman got two surrogates involved, and each of them delivered two babies" (Khazova 2013, 316-7). But the elderly lady could not be registered as the mother of any of them, as this is possible only for a married couple, so the babies live in a legal limbo.

for most [EU] Member States legal motherhood is attributed on the basis of parturition, irrespective of where the birth took place. Similar difficulties can arise in relation to legal fatherhood, as well as the recognition of two parents of the same sex. This can potentially leave a child not only legally parentless, but also stateless and without citizenship given that their birth registration documentation is not recognised beyond the country of birth. (European Parliament 2013, 10)

Intended parents probably do not think that they will be caught, but infants do get blocked at borders. Particularly dramatic was the case of Baby Manji, born in India, whose Japanese intended parents separated before her birth. The father wanted to recognize and bring home the baby, but India forbids single men to adopt female children. Plus, since the agreement was valid in India, Baby Manji was considered Japanese and could not acquire Indian nationality, but neither could she legally be bestowed with the Rising Sun nationality as her birth certificate was false for the Japanese authorities. Smerdon recounts other cases of "suspended babies." This looks like the most appalling of them: "An American woman created a stir when she left a baby at a passport office in Secunderabad on 25 January 2012 out of frustration at being unable to secure an Indian passport for the child who was born in December 2011" (Smerdon 2013, 215).

The problem of statelessness arises after the legal parenthood of the intended parents has been established in the state of birth (by original birth certificate, amended birth certificate, judicial decision, administration decree or adoption order) since to take the child out of that state, a passport or travel documentation must be issued. But embassies might not be able to recognize parenthood if the documents presented are contrary to *mater semper certa est*.

All of the cases risking statelessness—Baby Manji and the Balaz twins included—have been resolved by courts applying their arbitrary power of decision out of humanitarian reasons.[109] There is actually no known stateless child as a result of surrogacy agreements.[110] There is also a presumed need for the child to have legally defined parents—legal experts favorable to sur-

---

[109] See some solved cases in Trimmings and Beaumont 2013, 514 ff.). But there are no data: their survey on transnational surrogacy gave scant results due to nonparticipation of informants: just one intermediary described the 31 cases handled by him in the course of four and a half years (Trimmings and Beaumont 2013, 464 ff.).

[110] The last document by The Hague Conference, eager to recognize surrogacy contract, lists only a dozen of legal cases (*Private International Law Issues Surrounding The Status Of Children, Including Issues Arising From International Surrogacy Arrangements,* Document drawn up by the Permanent Bureau, March 2011).

rogacy contracts repeat this mantra for pushing their cause. Is it really the first need of a newborn? Again I must repeat myself: its interest is not to be separated from its mother. Once separated, the baby's needs change, and truly become not to be separated from the people who have taken care of it for some time (but we ignore how long it takes a newborn to forget its mother) even if they have broken the law. But to skip the very first passage is just a lawyer's trick.

A real problem infringing on the well-being of children is that the punishment for transgressing couples can be their separation from the child, as they are considered unfit parents because of the way they acquired parenthood—so the costs of implementing prohibitionist laws is borne (also) by the child, with another separation from its now *de facto* family (if they have taken care of it for some—undefined—time). There has been at least one case in Italy: a six-month-old child was taken away from its (by that time perhaps established) family to be placed in foster care. The decision of the Court for minors was upheld by Cassazione (the second and last appeal court, case 24001/ 2014): the baby was born in Ukraine with eggs from the surrogate mother and no genetic relationship to the intended father, which is also contrary to Ukrainian law and invalidates the birth certificate even there (case Paradiso and Campanelli, see further). A more recent development in Italy went against prohibitionism: the V Penal Section of the Tribunal in Milan on 15 October 2013 admitted the validity of a Ukrainian birth certificate as it was in accordance with the laws of that country. Then came the Mennesson case, establishing in 2014 a precedent for the whole EU, as we shall see.

In the meantime, *de facto* families, from a procedure that would be illegal at home, were in the end accepted also in Iceland,[111] in Germany by some tribunals (AG Nürnberg and LG Düsseldorf, see European Parliament 2013, 120 ff.), in Spain, where the parenthood of two men was recognized as it had the consent of the birth mother (European Parliament 2013, 125 ff), in Ireland, where in March 2013, the High Court ruled that the name of intended and genetic mother in a domestic surrogacy agreement should be put on the birth register, although it was in contrast with Irish law. Also Austria

---

[111] "Iceland Accepts Surrogate Baby Born in Thane," *Hindustan Times* 21.12.2010 http://www.hindustantimes.com/india--news/maharashtra/iceland--accepts--surrogate--baby--born--in--thane/article1--640934.aspx accessed 1.2.2015.

caved in, with a verdict of its Constitutional Court regarding two twins born in Ukraine: their birth certificate was validated in the best interest of the children, furthermore considering that it was impossible to force a woman who has given birth to act as a mother if she has refused to.[112] Other countries such as the Netherlands provide for a "partial recognition" of the birth certificate recognizing only the father listed in it. France had a rather complicated situation (European Parliament 2013, 114 ff.), that could be summed up in this way:

> the French refusal to issue a birth certificate has only a formal scope, without real impact on the daily lives of children who will have access to care and can go to school. One can also think that it would be possible to obtain a French identity card, on the basis of a French parentage bond established by a foreign certificate. Even in special situations, such as in cases of divorce or death of a parent, why would the judge or the notary, many years later, not be content with the foreign certificates without any suspicion about the circumstances of the birth of children? (European Parliament 2013, 117, on the basis of the interview Ms. Valérie Delnaud, Head of the Office of law of persons and family to the Directorate of Civil Affairs and the Seal, 26 March 2013)

But since 2014, the recognition of birth certificates that would be declared forged in the countries with *mater semper certa est*, is endorsed by the European Court of Human Right. The case Mennesson v. France was judged favorably to the petitioners under the principle of the protection of family life, inscribed in article 8 of the European Convention on Human Rights.[113] French authorities were compelled to validate birth certificates bearing the name of the intended mother (application no. 65192/11, analogous to Labassee v. France no. 65941/11). The petitioners were the Mennesson family, whose twin daughters, now 14-years-old, were born to a Californian woman. The (rare) fact that she had a higher income than the intended parents was recognized by the court as the proof that she made a true act of solidarity. It had already been recognized by French tribunals that the of-

---

[112] Cases *M.R & Anor v An tArd Chlaraitheoir & Ors*, [2013] IEHC 91), http://www.bailii.org/ie/cases/IEHC/2013/H91.html accessed 12.1.2015, and Verfassungsgerichtshof, 11.10.2012—B 99/12 ua.

[113] *Article 8: Right to respect for private and family life*.
1 Everyone has the right to respect for his private and family life, his home and his correspondence.
2. There shall be no interference by a public authority with the exercise of this right except such as is in accordance with the law and is necessary in a democratic society in the interests of national security, public safety or the economic wellbeing of the country, for the prevention of disorder or crime, for the protection of health or morals, or for the protection of the rights and freedoms of others.

fence of infringement of the status of the children was not punishable as committed outside French territory, so only the validity of the birth certificates was in question.[114]

The Mennesson's case established the recognition of families derived by surrogacy agreement in all EU member states, smiting France's opposition and its defense of *mater semper certa est*:

> [Point] 78. The Court observes in the present case that there is no consensus in Europe on the lawfulness of surrogacy arrangements or the legal recognition of the relationship between intended parents and children thus conceived abroad. A comparative-law survey conducted by the Court shows that surrogacy is expressly prohibited in fourteen of the thirty-five member States of the Council of Europe—other than France—studied. In ten of these it is either prohibited under general provisions or not tolerated, or the question of its lawfulness is uncertain. However, it is expressly authorized in seven member States and appears to be tolerated in four others. In thirteen of these thirty-five States it is possible to obtain legal recognition of the parent-child relationship between the intended parents and the children conceived through a surrogacy agreement legally performed abroad.
> This also appears to be possible in eleven other States (including one in which the possibility may only be available in respect of the father-child relationship where the intended father is the biological father), but excluded in the eleven remaining States (except perhaps the possibility in one of them of obtaining recognition of the father-child relationship where the intended father is the biological father). [...]
> 79. This lack of consensus reflects the fact that recourse to a surrogacy arrangement raises sensitive ethical questions. It also confirms that the States must in principle be afforded a wide margin of appreciation, regarding the decision not only whether or not to authorize this method of assisted reproduction but also whether or not to recognise a legal parent-child relationship between children legally conceived as the result of a surrogacy arrangement abroad and the intended parents.
> 80. However, regard should also be had to the fact that an essential aspect of the identity of individuals is at stake where the legal parent-child relationship is concerned. The margin of appreciation afforded to the respondent State in the present case therefore needs to be reduced. (Case of Mennesson v. France. Application no. 65192/11)

The European Court deliberated on 15th January 2015 that the case Paradiso and Campanelli v. Italy constituted another violation of article 8 of the European Convention on Human Rights. This is the story:

---

[114] The norms against surrogacy are only valid in French territory. In France not only civil status is inalienable, but it is a penal offence to incite to abandon a born or unborn child "either for pecuniary gain, or by gifts, promises, threats or abuse of authority." It is also forbidden "acting for pecuniary gain as an intermediary between a person desiring to adopt a child and a parent desiring to abandon its born or unborn child" (art. 227-12 of the Penal Code), including a woman agreeing to bear a child with the intent to give it up.

> A surrogacy contract was agreed between an Italian couple and a Russian company, "Rosjurconsulting." A child was born from a Russian woman. The birth certificate states that the child is the son of the Italian couple of intent. Upon their return to Italy, the parents asked to have the birth certificate transcribed, but the Italian administration (Ufficiale di Stato civile) refused to do so under the premise that the birth certificate did not state the name of the real parents.
>
> It dealt with a very special case of surrogacy, because neither the intended father nor the intended mother were the genetic parents of the child born through the Russian woman. Biological tests were indeed carried out.
>
> This couple avoided not only the ban on reproduction with gametes from donors, but the rules about the adoption too. The Court for minors had to declare a state of abandon (and adoptability) regarding the child, because the biological parents were unknown and the intended parents could not be considered parents—according to Italian law—without any genetic or legal ties to the minor. The Court refused to foster the child to the intended parents. The judgment denying the foster is related to the discretion of the judges, as it is generally employed in the Italian Court of minors. The Court of Appeal confirmed the first judgment. The child was entrusted to the social services and placed in foster care. The couple has no contact with him. (European Parliament 2013, 125)

The "suspended babies" condition is pitiful, and tribunals who break established family ties are ruthless (the baby was declared adoptable when six months old), but how should courts defend the laws of their country? Ignorance of the law must be fought against to prevent similar cases. But apart from the case above and a few similar ones, courts are generally reluctant to punish intended parents. Could it be because, as rich people, they are considered above the law?

> There was no mention of prosecuting the Sterns for breaking the law, even though the court maintained that theirs was a serious crime, punishable by 3–5 years in prison. In some sense, the Sterns were rewarded for breaking the law through custody of "Baby M." (Oliver 1989 103)

International conventions muddle the matter instead of clarifying it, as they only apparently proscribe the sale of children. The Convention on the Rights of the Child (1989) forbids cross-border movements derived from the sale of children even if the aim is purely to have a family: "States Parties shall take all appropriate national, bilateral and multilateral measures to prevent the abduction of, the sale of or traffic in children for any purpose or in any form" (art. 35). The Hague Convention on Protection of Children and Co-Operation in Respect of Intercountry Adoption (1993)—not a UN document but signed by 89 countries, including India, China and all Southern America countries (not the US)—establishes the same principle: "the consents [to adoption] have not been induced by payment or compensation of any kind" (art. 4), and "the consent of the mother, where required, has been given only after the birth of required legal form, and expressed or evidenced in writing" (art. 5). Plus, it must be verified that "the child is or will be authorized to enter and reside permanently in that State."

But both Conventions in reality forbid "improper gains" (art. 8 of the Hague Convention, while art. 21 of the Convention on the Rights of the Child forbids "improper financial gain" in intercountry adoption). This expression might only mean that gain is improper, that improperness is the reason why gains are forbidden, but it is generally interpreted to mean that—while "improper" gains are forbidden—other kind of gains are admitted. From this perspective, the jurist Yasmine Ergas has tried to disentangle the matter, starting from the fact that: "There is an evident trend in international law towards the prohibition of the sale of persons *no matter what their status either prior or subsequent to the sale itself* (Ergas 2012a, 88). Then Ergas counterbalances this line of reasoning quoting the work of Viviane Zelizer (1985), who demonstrated the normalcy of intermeshing "love and money," which is a fact of life in a capitalist context (though it must be noticed that in her preeminent historical analysis of adoption practices, the point of view of the birth mother on the commercialization of their babies is totally disregarded). Ergas concludes drawing a line in the sand by allowing "proper compensation." The reason of her indecisiveness is that both conventions suggest "that some measure of gain may be legitimate" (Ergas 2012a, 89, see also Ergas 2013).

Despite the rhetorical engagement of states against markets for babies, the little word "improper" is now made to legitimize a sale of children in adoption—and in surrogacy if the situation is deemed analogous—but only a sale that does not bring a lot of profit to its various actors. This, as Ergas writes, has created a slippery slope in adoption analogous to the "reimbursement of foregone gains" in surrogacy:

> recent reviews of the implementation of the Convention acknowledge that such payments [for reasonable expenses] often function as surreptitious forms of compensation for the transfer of parental rights. The Secretary of the Hague Conference on Private International Law has noted: "The connection between money and intercountry adoption is a fact of life and it is better to acknowledge that and try to regulate it."[115]

---

[115] Jennifer Degeling, *The Intercountry Adoption to Good Practice Revisited: Good practice and real practice*, Hague Conference on Private International Law, Nordic Adoption Council Meeting, 2009, 4-5th November, 2009, Rejkavik, Iceland (quoted by Ergas 2012a, 83 n. 215).

This is the climate in which the possibility of an international surrogacy convention will be considered. The Hague Conference has in fact been asked to draft a proposal, after New Zealand requested it to evaluate whether its Convention on Adoption of 1993 might be applied to international surrogacy cases. The answer was negative. To date, three documents[116] have been produced from the point of view of the states which admit the contract and establish parent-child relationships without *mater semper certa est*. The problem then becomes to have these contracts recognized, remedying the ignorance of the law (or the bad faith) of the couples travelling abroad to obtain a child through this procedure (what the experts call "recognition of parenthood"). Let us hope that the discussion will further progress before a Convention is proposed.

Finally, law-breaking happens in places where contracts are fully legal, as in California, too:

> a US lawyer, for example, created an inventory of available babies by exporting American gestational carriers to Ukraine, where they were impregnated with sperm from anonymous donors. When the pregnancies reached the second trimester, the lawyer offered the future children to clients for $100,000, presenting them as the products of surrogacy contracts that had fallen through. (Ergas 2012a, 76–7 n 187[117])

This is not the only case of "malpractice." Another California lawyer, Andrew Vorzimer, is advocating for regulation, licensing and oversight on what he calls the Wild West of California surrogacy: "I've been practicing in this field for two decades [...] In the last three years I've seen more scandals and ethical deviations than anything I'd witness in the previous 17 years" (Thompson 2013, 16). This might have something to do with the increasing popularity of surrogacy, and the growth of foreign demand: in short, with the normalization of getting babies in this way. The most problematic cases he recounts show a preoccupying trend in the intended parents' attitude:

---

[116] See *The private international law issues surrounding the status of children, including issues arising from international surrogacy arrangements*. Key documents (http://www.hcch.net/index_en.php?act=text.display&tid=178 accessed 13.1.2015).

[117] Original note: "California Lawyer Ordered to Prison in Baby Scam," *The Tennessean*, 25 February 2012, [no more] available at: http://www.tennessean.com/article/20120225/NEWS08/302250066/California-lawyer-ordered-prison-baby-selling-scam.

> One man, he recalls, asked him to arrange for a surrogate to carry a half-dozen of his embryos, since he wanted at least quadruplets. Not so he could raise all of those babies, the man said, but so he could choose the best one and put the rest up for adoption. "I didn't know what to say," Vorzimer recalls. "Eventually I stammered, "What are you looking for, the pick of the litter?" And he said, "That's exactly what I'm looking for."[118] [...] One international couple, upon learning the fetus was not the gender they had hoped for, threatened to withhold medical compensation from their surrogate unless she aborted. Another couple tried to put their vanity baby up for adoption because it was born prematurely. (Thompson 2013, 16)

But all this would be perfectly legal. Then there are the law-breaking cases of agencies disappearing with the money, as SurroGenesis did in 2009, informing its closure by email to about 100 intended parents and surrogates, never to give back the 2.5 million USD that it held in "trust accounts." Regulation is sometimes asked for only to control the behavior of agencies (but with or without regulation of agencies, surrogacy contracts are already legalization of baby-selling):

> According to Hanafin [psychologist for the Center for Surrogate Parenting of Los Angeles], the worst problems stemmed from the rise of surrogacy agents. These are the unlicensed go-betweens who introduce intended parents to the surrogates, coordinate with doctors and psychotherapists to screen the parties for infectious disease and mental health problems, find lawyers to draw up the contracts, and oversee escrow accounts set up to fund surrogacy fees and expenses.
> It's a tough job, requiring knowledge of medicine and the law, attention to detail, and a keen appreciation that you're responsible for the health and future of other human beings. Hanafin claims that a growing number of lazy, incompetent, or unscrupulous people represent themselves as agents with no more bona fides than a laptop computer. (Thompson 2013, 19)

There is another kind of suspended baby: those who are rejected because they are handicapped. The advocates of surrogacy always underline this situation as the basis for the necessity of a contract, in order not to have the birth mother "stuck" with a baby she did not intend to rear, as if she were compelled by law to do so. Only in this case do they take for granted moth-

---

[118] This is not the only example: "In April 1988, surrogate mother Patty Nowakowski gave birth to fraternal twins, a boy and a girl. The couple which had contracted for Mrs. Nowakowski's services as a surrogate mother refused to accept the baby boy, giving as a reason that they already had three male children and they did not want another. They were willing, however, to accept, and did take custody of, the baby girl. Mrs. Nowakowski sent the rejected baby boy to a foster home, but she later changed her mind and reclaimed him, deciding that she would raise him herself. About six weeks later Mrs. Nowakowski also reclaimed the baby girl by refusing to consent to her adoption by the contracting couple." (Krimmel 1992, 8. Original reference: "Rejected Boy's Twin Also With Mother," L.A. Times, 29.5.1988, http://articles.latimes.com/1988-05-29/news/mn-5294_1_twin-boys-mother accessed 21.1.2015).

erly love and the emotional impossibility of a birth mother to relinquish her child to adoption. I must however admit that, at least in one case, the pressure on the intended parents from having signed a contract worked:

> In one case, a child was born with "an apparent hearing loss." The intended parents, a French couple, were "nervous about receiving the child" as they perceived that "there was not great support for deaf children in France." Nevertheless, after being advised by Participant 1 [an interviewed "broker"], who explained the details of their obligations under the surrogacy contract and the responsibility as the legal parents in the eyes of the relevant US law, they willingly took the child home and are currently raising it. (Trimmings and Beaumont 2013, 480)

But there are many other cases where the intended parents just didn't.[119]

National laws can be circumvented by cross-border movements of people who have the resources to do it—and it is more and more just a question of money, as information can easily be accessed from the internet, where clinics advertise in many languages. This is lamented as class discrimination (or rather as a discrimination based on money, as the c-word has dis-

---

[119] And a few horror stories as well. Murder: "a single man 'commissioned' a genetically-related child through a traditional surrogacy agreement in Pennsylvania. The baby, however, died six weeks after the birth as a result of physical abuse" (*Huddleston v Infertility Clinic of America Inc*, 20 August 1997, in Trimming and Beaumont 2013, 529 n. 314).
Things happening in India: "Eg. the story of a 22-year-old, Kavita Rakesh, who, due to pressing financial problems her family was facing, took a heartbreaking decision to abort her own baby to become a surrogate mother (F. Eliot, "Only Baby Couple Can Afford Is a Stranger's," *The Times* 10 April 2012, http://www.thetimes.co.uk/tto/news/world/asia/article3379054.ece accessed 28,12,2014, a similar story in Pande 2014, 114).
Death: "Eg. the story of a 30-year-old surrogate mother, Pamela Vaghels, who died in an Ahmedabad hospital in May 2012 during a routine check-up after delivering a baby for American intended parents: *The New Indian Time Express*, 14 June 2012, available at www.newindianexpress.com/editorials/article542128.ece" (Trimming and Beaumont 2013, 529 n. 311).
Unscrupulous birth mothers: "Eg. the Belgian case of *Baby D*. Court of Appeal, Ghent, 5 September 2005, where a Belgian surrogate entered into a surrogacy agreement with a Belgian couple. The surrogate later informed the couple that she had miscarried, whilst 'selling' the baby to a Dutch couple she had met online" (Trimming and Beaumont 2013, 529 n. 315).
The selling of fetuses (mentioned above): "A renowned California lawyer and a surrogate mom each got hit with jail time Friday for their roles in a black market operation that sold unborn fetuses to prospective parents for upwards of $100,000. Surrogacy attorney Theresa Erickson and repeat surrogate Carla Chambers had faced the possibility of five years behind bars, but both ultimately received just five months in federal custody along with subsequent stints of house arrest. Prosecutors said the women promised candidates to be surrogate mothers for up to $45,000 each to travel to the Ukraine and be implanted with fertilized embryos that would then be offered for sale during the third trimester" (Dillon 2012).

appeared from contemporary vocabulary), and again legalization is proposed as the solution—though surrogacy contracts not only imply expenditure at home as well, but also the division between those who can afford commissioning a baby and those women who will sell their procreative capacity because of economic necessity. The freedom to buy and sell babies will look a lot like the splendid freedom to sleep under bridges, equally accessible to the rich and to the poor. But, contrary to the advantages of sleeping in the open for the poor, it is the rich who will take advantage of a baby market, legally forcing women to give up their children out of economic necessity.

Human rights of surrogacy babies

Yasmine Ergas has examined the question whether existing human rights laws would require either a prohibition or an acceptance of transnational surrogacy, which she identifies with commercial surrogacy because no element of solidarity can subsist between strangers across borders. As Ergas finds arguments both in favor and against prohibition of surrogacy, she does not give a definite answer to the question that she finds fundamental: whether or not the "best interest of the child" principle calls for a permissive stance towards the regulation of surrogacy. On one hand, prohibitionism might create stateless children (an argument that I find weak and specious), on the other, the *habeas corpus* of the surrogate mother would not be respected by the protection of surrogacy contracts. She inconclusively concludes that violations of human rights would occur either by international prohibition or by a legalization of surrogacy.

But, she recalls, in international conventions the sale of children in adoption is prohibited only if an "improper" gain is obtained. Commodification, she writes, has also tainted international adoption, and it stems mainly from the combination of economic inequalities with a strong "demand" for adoption from rich countries. As this demand cannot be satisfied by the number of existing orphans, monetary incentives are offered to the poor to abandon their children. Analysts as Susan Markens (2007) have shown how both international adoption and surrogacy *are* markets in human beings, and: "There can be little doubt that the commodification of human beings runs counter to the primary thrust of contemporary international human rights law" (Ergas 2013, 327). But again the proposal is to avoid "improper" gains.

What Ergas leaves out of her analysis is the importance of the human right guaranteeing family life: this is the human right that mother and newborn should enjoy. In my view, the question whether surrogacy contracts violate human rights should be framed in terms of the pressure they put on birth mothers to abandon their children, whether by monetary restitutions or by "specific performance," with the force of the state separating mother and child: clearly a violation of the human right to "family life."

The continuity of family life, sanctioned by international conventions such as the Convention on the Rights of the Child (1989) and the Hague Convention on Protection of Children and Co-operation in Respect of Intercountry Adoption (1993), is a powerful reason why there cannot be a right to reproduce through a(nother) woman. The Convention on the Rights of the Child says: "The child [...] shall have [...]. as far as possible, the right to know and be cared for by his or her parents."[120] And in the preamble of the Hague Convention the parties are "recalling that each State should take, as a matter of priority, appropriate measures to enable the child to remain in the care of his or her family of origin." If a woman who has given birth cannot raise her baby out of economic difficulties, states have even pledged to help the child maintain its familial ties, and logically this can only mean financial help to the mother in order for her not to abandon the child. Admittedly, in a non-Finemanian universe, the concept of "family" is itself unclear. So how is the right to grow up with one's family to be interpreted? Even in a non-Finemanian universe, at birth this can only mean the tie with the mother, with the birth mother. So there is no reason in terms of internationally agreed or constitutional rights why she should renounce her baby if she does not really want to.

Ergas also mentions the possibility that the "right to work" could be relevant for adopting a stance, again without affirming it with certainty. It is not a moot point how the "work" of the surrogate is conceptualized by those who want to validate contracts: is she giving gestational services, so that her right to work is exercised or, given that she is not going to be part

---

[120] The whole text of art. 7, paragraph 1, is: "The child shall be registered immediately after birth and shall have the right from birth to a name, the right to acquire a nationality and as far as possible, the right to know and be cared for by his or her parents" (in fact, the estimation of unregistered babies in the world is 50 million). But this Convention has not been ratified by the US, "the world's greatest importer of foreign born children" (Bartner 2000, 425).

of its family, is she selling her baby, an act which is internationally forbidden (according to commentators), outside cases of adoption "with proper gains"? If this is the case, if the surrogate's job is just to give "gestational services," John Stuart Mill and the liberal point of view would be satisfied, as both Hatzis and the Report to the European Parliament recall: "Mill's principle that only harmful practices [to others, of course, but the language of the Report is sloppy] should be prohibited by law and that one is ultimately sovereign over one's body and mind" (European Parliament 2013, 23). But this Millean principle applied to pregnancy should—at its minimum—entail that the surrogate is sovereign over the future baby, as long as it is a part of her body. What does it exactly mean to apply it afterwards? And is it a "harmful practice" for the child if a woman "leases" her body and has somebody else's baby? There are two kinds of answers: a legal one and a biological one—which Marvin Harris would have called an answer reflecting the culture that is being studied and an answer describing the observations made in the most objective way possible on behavior and actions. This is the answer given by a supporter of baby markets:

> In the context of the gestational agreement, the embryo belongs to its parents. We cannot speak of baby-selling, since the surrogate cannot sell something she does not have: i.e., parental rights to the newborn. The surrogate is essentially selling her labor, her gestational services. (Hatzis 2009, 209)

This echoes a testimony by a surrogate mother reported by the anthropologist Gillian Goslinga-Roy:

> Whenever accused of 'baby selling, which was fairly often, she would confidently retort, "How can I sell a baby which is not mine in the first place? I'm not genetically related to this child. It is not mine to sell!" (Goslinga-Roy 2000, 117)

These answers mainly employ juridical concepts (Marx would say superstructural, ideological): "parental rights," "property of an embryo" or of a child, cultural concepts that have nothing to do with the biological processes of pregnancy and birth. The surrogate mother also uses a legitimation of "property" based on genetics and not on pregnancy, which is also a cultural and not a biological trait, if used to trump the role of pregnancy. In fact the lawyers' reasoning stands or falls only from the legal definition of the action itself: if the baby belongs to its genetic parents, the surrogate is indeed providing a service, if the child belongs to her (as she is the one who made it, as argued in the first chapter and as commonsense dictates) then she is legally selling it. Hatzis' reasoning (and Shalev before him) already implies that the embryo belongs to the genetic contributors, the male and female fathers, so the surrogate mother can be seen as working, giving them gestational services. But this begs the question, we can say that she is selling her gestational services only if we already believe that she is not entitled to any parental right. Lawyers notwithstanding, she is the mother both by biology and under *mater semper certa est* (in most states, where it still exists). Life does not recognize property, much less property in embryos.

But even if we conceded that the surrogate mother exercises a right to work, there is no right "to perform whatever kind of work in whatsoever conditions offered." Quite the contrary: the collective action by workers carves out rights *not* to work in whatsoever conditions, posing limits to hours and kind of activity, requiring protection for health, a minimum hourly pay and benefits. "Work" is not an abstract and undefined concept but a very concrete one, articulated in tasks and conditions, and its content depends on the class struggle between the entrepreneurs (or the state), and the workers. There is no "right" to access to types and conditions of work that have been excluded by collective bargaining, as it would only mean underselling one's labor power and provoking collective damage for a personal benefit. To go beyond the legal limits posed for concrete work is not "to exercise free choice" but to worsen the collective position of the working class—a position which of course is complicated by national borders and by the rules and bargaining power peculiar to working in each country or zone—as shown by the tragedy of the establishment of the Export Processing Zones, created to attract capital by forfeiting on taxes and allowing it to exploit workers and natural resources on "exceptional" conditions.

So the question of regulating surrogacy by recognizing the surrogate's activity as work could in theory find a different solution in different states, but practically if the borders are kept open by the recognition of foreign contracts, this means a race to the bottom towards Indian conditions. The question of the admissibility of gestation as labor is equivalent to a loss of collective labor rights for all women also outside the poorest countries (with good private health care, without which no surrogacy arrangement can be credibly marketed) and depends on a change of the "public mind," that would render baby-buying a socially acceptable way to become parents. At present, intended parents who are shopping for a baby are relatively few, but with the spread of the practice normalization occurs, pushing the collective position of women clearly back in terms of concrete rights as workers: it will be considered acceptable to sell not just an external performance, but something happening within a woman's body, day and night, with all the pain and danger bound-up with gestation. Then finally the birth mother would be routinely forced to detach from her newborn and to consider what has happened to her body as an alien invasion by someone else's property, even being liable for damage to the fetus, and having to repress the emotions of becoming a mother. This was the condition of pregnant slaves: surrogacy contracts that are upheld by law are reminiscent of the practices slave owners imposed on Black women. Sadly, this is the situation described for Israel by Elly Teman (2010). Pregnancy can certainly be considered a job, but its incidence on personal relationships and on the sovereignty over one's body is unheard of in any other kind of employment (not even in violent professional sports, not even in prostitution: they are not a continuous invasion of the body for the duration of nine months). Transformation of pregnancy into a job, opening a market to sell reproductive capacities, implies a much diminished (or low, to start with) contractual power of women as a class. Of course the establishment of a labor market for services which, before that, were performed as duties *is* progress: Paola Tabet has shown that in a number of cultures alive before the expansion of the monetary circuit of D-M-D', the reproductive capacity of women was appropriated by men with collective violence. But in capitalist countries belonging to the core this is not so clear anymore: procreative decisions are shared in couples, and women decide even independently to become mothers—though social pressure to reproduce is still an important cultural trait. We can say that social reproduction is guaranteed by ideological factors, but an element of female choice and freedom is guaranteed. To start selling reproductive capacities that women have begun to exercise independently does not seem like much progress. Nor is it a question of "respecting agency," as this is not the only parameter to avail decisions about work. The Appeal Court in New Jersey which judged the Baby M case spelled it out in clear letters:

> The point is made that Mrs. Whitehead [the surrogate] *agreed* to the surrogacy arrangement, supposedly fully understanding the consequences. Putting aside the issue of how compelling her need for money may have been, and how significant her understanding of the consequences, we suggest that her consent is irrelevant. There are, in a civilized society, some things that money cannot buy. In America, we decided long ago that merely because conduct purchased by money was "voluntary " did not mean that it was good or beyond regulation and prohibition. *West Coast Hotel Co. v. Parrish*, 300 US 379, 57 *S.Ct.* 578, 81 *L.Ed.* 703 (1937). Employers can no longer buy labor at the lowest price they can bargain for, even though that labor is "voluntary, " 29 *USC.* ß 206 (1982), or buy women's labor for less money than paid to men for the same job, 29 *USC.* ß 206(d), or purchase the agreement of children to perform oppressive labor, 29 *USC.* ß 212, or purchase the agreement of workers to subject themselves to unsafe or unhealthful working conditions, 29 *USC.* §§ 651 to 678. (Occupational Safety and Health Act of 1970). There are, in short, values that society deems more important than granting to wealth whatever it can buy, be it labor, love, or life. Whether this principle recommends prohibition of surrogacy, which presumably sometimes results in great satisfaction to all of the parties, is not for us to say. We note here only that, under existing law, the fact that Mrs. Whitehead "agreed " to the arrangement is not dispositive (*In the Matter of Baby M*, 537 A.2d 1227, N.J. 1988)

And it is not for me to say how collective women's position in India can be improved—but certainly not by selling "womb products" for the internal market and for export. To answer the Supreme Court of New Jersey, I personally do not want to prohibit generosity, but generosity cannot be compelled by contract or by economic menace. Also Martha Field feared the creation of such a class of breeders:

> Laws prohibiting surrogacy *are* protectionist toward women, but they also accord best with the kind of society we want to live in. A common attack against those who would ban surrogacy is that they are advocating legislation for women in an ideal world, whereas women in the real world need these opportunities and should be able to take advantage of them. But to portray surrogacy contracts as representing meaningful choice and informed consent on the part of the contracting surrogate mother, rather than to see her as driven by circumstances, also reveals an idealized perspective and a failure to take account of realities. (Field 1988, 27)

Moreover, and settling the issue, pregnancy is not the kind of job a woman can lay claim to by virtue of her right to work, as it entails not just the selling of her service, but the selling of her child, in relation to which she carries maternal rights and duties being its birth mother (I cannot think of a more "natural right" than to keep caring for one's newborn). Commodification may not always be a bad thing for women trapped in the patriarchal domestic mode of production, but there must be other ways to make a living that do not create a market for babies. Even if individual women can thrive by occasionally taking part in it, the institution is repugnant.

In places where surrogacy is already considered as work, as in India (where cosmetic reasons are advanced to deny it), the stigmatization of this activity, seen as an extramarital pregnancy involving sexual infidelity, guarantees at the moment a high compensation for the few women and families willing to do it. At the time of Pande's ethnography the intended parents were queueing up at the clinics. If surrogacy becomes normalized, demand for babies will grow, but the offer of wombs to rent will grow much more in this context of poverty, with the likely result of a drop in income towards the level of retribution of any other unskilled labor.

Another controversial question that applies to surrogacy is whether there is a right to know one's origin. The child's curiosity, or "need" (in inverted commas as it is socially determined, see the works of Barbara Katz Rothman) to know its origin despite the fact that neither genetic contributions nor the birth mother did really want to father or to mother it, has already been called a right to know one's origin, though the question is much debated. At best it can be a right under conditions. In international law the matter is ambiguous: article 7 of the Convention of the Rights of the Child establishes for the child "as far as possible, the right to know and be cared for by his or her parents" without mentioning weather information about them must be conserved when they are *de facto* not in its family. The European Human Rights Court struck a balance between the child's right to know who its parents are and the parent's right to privacy. The two rights are clearly conflicting and, as in adoption, neither can prevail: the wisest thing to do in surrogacy would be to keep records of eventual donors and of the birth mother, accessible with a request for contact by the person concerned.

A child has perhaps a moral right to know his or her origin, to be fulfilled with the moral duty by its parents to inform it (with the help of public registries), but this rather seems just another matter for which (social) parents are responsible, and that is sometimes resolved in a way that differs from what the child itself would have preferred. Again, as the child has a dependent status, it must accept many parental decisions, including the anonymity of its gamete contributors.

We must also notice that other states' rules are very important in the decision of single women and lesbian couples about anonymity: the rules governing the genetic contributors' possible intromission into their family.

Many lesbian couples or single women decide in favor of anonymity because they fear a paternity suit by a man whom they do not need nor want in the upbringing of their children. Phyllis Chesler (among others) noted that if a sperm donor changes his mind (men are always allowed a change of heart, she writes), the courts in the US will most certainly recognize him as the legal father, complete with visitation or even custody rights, especially if the mother is not under any "reproductive contract" with a man.

Nevertheless organizations of adopted children have fought for this right to know, for "open adoption" that preserves data and contact details about their genetic mother/parents. The historical reason for anonymity of birth mothers was that they wouldn't want to let anybody know their shame for the pregnancy—which involved extramarital sex. So to be able to forget the baby and the shame, they shouldn't be reminded of its existence. But birth mothers do look for their adopted children, and viceversa. Both are especially outraged when forbidden to access information that does exist in state archives. Now a movement of donor-conceived persons is campaigning for the same right to know their origin. This could, and perhaps should, be influential on the intended parent(s) decision, not only in cases of surrogacy but in general, without introducing an absolute right to know one's origin. The reason is that, besides children from anonymous gametes, there are children conceived with a sexual relationship between strangers, or in adultery. These conceptions have happened, and always will—so the principle of truth and disclosure about everybody's origin cannot be considered a basic human right: some families would be destroyed by its application. The European Court of Human Rights deliberated in fact that the rights to privacy and to the integrity of family life trump an hypothetical "right to know" the actual truth about one's origin.

The countries that have instituted a legal right to this knowledge, have never obliged the biological contributors to meet up with their offspring—they could in fact never enforce that. They just take upon themselves the duty to store the information about their whereabouts, making a request for contact possible, for example in the Netherlands at the 16th birthday of the child, or at the 25th in Italy. The authorities in charge forward the message, but whether the meeting with one's genetic parent(s) will take place is a matter of willingness.

Some states have affirmed such a right to the knowledge of one's origin, and/or prohibited the anonymous donation of gametes, such as Sweden and Venezuela. In New Zealand "donor offspring should be made aware of their genetic origins and be able to access information about those origins" when they turn 18.[121] Anonymity of genetic contributors was eliminated in the Netherlands in 2004 and in the UK in 2005, and this has had the interesting and perhaps foreseeable consequence that the number of "donors" dramatically decreased. But not all the citizens are convinced of the good of the norm, and many couples cross borders towards neighboring lands to enjoy donor anonymity. Not only surrogacy rules can prescribe the traceability of gamete contributors and surrogate mothers, as in the UK, but the right to personal identity can encompass the right to know one's origin, as in Israel:

> the Embryo Carrying Agreement Ordinance 1998 creates a registry in which all successful surrogacy procedures are registered. The registry must contain the names and details of the child, surrogate and intended parents, as well as details of the court case and any orders made by the court regarding future relationships between the parties. All changes and updates must also be submitted to the registrar. This registry is not open to the public; however, when a person born through surrogacy reaches his or her majority (18 years), he or she may obtain a social worker's permission to see the record. A social worker's refusal to grant access to the record may be contested in court. (Shakargy 2013, 241)

Nevertheless, the law in the making does not seem to be so favorable to the requests of children of donors or adoptees to know their origin. India's Draft Bill on surrogacy, introduced already in 2010 and not yet approved, would require the anonymity of gamete donors and birth mothers. Some countries recently introduced "safe haven" laws allowing for anonymous delivery in order to reduce infanticide. In South Africa, the Children's Act peculiarly established a right to know one's origins comprising only physical description, not identity, unless the donors agree to leave contact data. For surrogacy, this matter must be settled in the agreement, where the future contact between the surrogate and her child is detailed (Slabbert and Roodt 2013, 342).

The overwhelming importance that the law assumes at the moment of the detachment of the birth mother from her child has now been highlight-

---

[121] S. 4 (c) of the Human Assisted Reproductive Technology Act 2004 (quoted by Achmad 2013, 297 and 300).

ed—though it is true that in many places the rule of law is just an illusion, and the concrete relations of power and inequality substantially strip the socially weakest classes and genders of all rights. Surrogates in India are told very little about their pregnancy (e.g. often they do not know how many babies they are carrying), let alone be able to decide about its outcome. Vietnamese women have been kidnapped and raped to be used as captured wombs in Thailand.[122] In Mexico, India, Russia, but also the US, agencies are cheating the intended parents, taking their money without any intention to deliver any child, and in Russia individual surrogates do the same.[123] TV news and documentaries have shown us the indifferent faces of some of the culprits, together with the desperate looks of surrogate mothers who can not afford another child to rear, who discovered that the clinic for which they worked had disappeared. So they were basically knocked up and abandoned by their doctors and agents.

---

[122] ABC News. *Women freed from 'inhuman' baby ring*, 25 February 2011 (http://www.abc.net.au/news/stories/2011/02/25/3148396.htm?section¼world accessed 27 November 2012). "In February 2010 the police arrested a Taiwanese brokering agency called 'Baby 101' and held in custody 15 Vietnamese women who were being trafficked to deliver 'designer babies' to foreign clients for a fee of about USD3,000" (Hibino and Shimazono 2013, 57).

[123] From a forum: "Circumstances have left me at 27 years old unable to have children. My husband hasn't left me (and for that, an enormous thank you to him). We decided to use the services of a surrogate mother and ran into a host of problems beyond nightmares. They cheat, come to you already pregnant, etc. They all have unimaginable fees: a one room apartment in Petersburg, $40–60,000. The surrogate mothers' logic is understandable—'I'm giving birth to a baby for you, giving it to you, so put me in luxury.' We can't afford this kind of sum. For that reason I'm addressing the applicants: DON'T CREATE ARTIFICIAL DEMAND. Two years ago the services costs $5,000. Have prices risen in these two years 10–15 times? Please share your experiences so we can figure out this problem."(Rivkin-Fish 2013, 579).

Chapter 4)
Mothers and others

The subjective experience

We can now look at how women are living through fertilization, pregnancy, and birth in a surrogacy agreement, and what the social meanings attributed to these life-passages resulting in the creation a new human life by surrogate mothers are. I have preferred to call them "birth mothers" because not only the pregnancy, but also the preparation of the mother's body to lactate in order to nourish the infant is obviously the same with or without a surrogacy agreement, no matter whether they think that the baby is theirs or not.[124] This is the body. What about the mind? The dichotomy is of course not precise, as the mind is an expression of the body and expresses itself through it: the intentional interaction of the pregnant woman with the fetus also includes physical interaction. Some surrogates hardly touch their swelling belly, fearing that they will start feeling a connection to the baby that will make their separation from it difficult, and some did not lactate immediately after delivery, but only days after (Teman 2010, 86). Surrogate mothers basically affirm that they are bearing a baby with whom they don't have a maternal relationship, and in most cases this is enough to guarantee a smooth process in fulfilling their promise (but see further the role of agencies in structuring this experience). It is not even a matter of being a gestational surrogate: genes are surely determinant for some women, who would never carry a child conceived with their own eggs (all of the Israelis for example), but not for others, who leave the choice whether to become a traditional or

---

[124] Except that it seems that surrogate pregnancies are more difficult. Even Elly Teman, who extolls surrogacy as valuable work, compares its uneasiness (testified by surrogates who claim a worse experience of pregnancy than with their own children) with the deteriorating health of other dispossessed: "Coker interprets the illness narratives of Sudanese refugees in Egypt as somatic testimonials to their political powerlessness and the loss of their land and community. Since the same pattern of symptoms and interpretations occurred among surrogates who conceived on 'natural' cycles without hormones and among those who were medically prepared for conception, I would suggest that the surrogates, like the refugees, are expressing a type of somatic and narrative resistance to their situation" (Teman 2010, 45).

a gestational surrogate to the intended parents (though they might be the minority).[125]

Compared to the number that went well, few are the cases of known litigation about the delivery of babies and also few the cases of other conflicts between surrogate mothers and intended parents reported in the press.[126] The British lawyer Natalie Gamble observes in an article entitled "Should surrogate mothers still have an absolute right to change their minds?" ("No" is her answer):

> Over the past 20 years, we have seen nearly 1,000 parental orders granted in the UK, with only two reported cases of the surrogate seeking to keep the baby. In one, the court gave residence to the intended parents; in the other, the surrogate mother—both decisions were made on a best interests basis given the particular facts. (Gamble 2012)

But litigation in the UK is necessary only if the birth mother first relinquished the child and then regretted it. The non-profit British agency COTS (Childlessness Overcome Though Surrogacy) reports that 2% of their agreements ended with the birth mothers keeping their children (Phillips 2013, 89) while, earlier on, the Brazier report estimated the unsuccessful arrangement at 4–5% (Brazier, Campbell and Golombok 1998, 26). But if out of a number of human interactions only a few entail violence, is it a good reason to dismiss them? There is little doubt that a forced separation of the birth mother from her child is an act of cruelty: why should it be considered acceptable to exercise it only for a small percentage of surrogate mothers? And if it seems that women who regret the separation are the exceptions to the norm, the true norm in fact is constituted by all the other women who would never dream of getting into this kind of agreement. A surrogate mother herself objects to the portrayal of surrogacy as an easy thing to do: "I started having doubts as soon as I was pregnant. They had these girls on TV saying how easy it was and how good it made them feel, but nobody

---

[125] A Facebook remark on the current scarcity of traditional surrogates in Britain: "As an IP [intended parent] I always think the deciding factor for a surro would be his you [her?] feel about the drugs for GS [gestational surrogacy] or the biology of carrying a child that is technically yours? There do seem to be less TS [traditional surrogates] around at the moment though."

[126] E.g. Caroline Graham: "Surrogate fathers tore my life apart: Used abused and called trailer trash...how UK poster boys for gay fatherhood turned on woman hired for her womb," *Mail Online* (*Daily Mail*), 3.1.2015. http://www.dailymail.co.uk/femail/article-2895772/Surrogate-fathers-tore-life-apart-Used-abused-called-trailer-trash-UK-poster-boys-gay-fatherhood-turned-woman-hired-womb.html?ito=social-facebook accessed 2.2.2015.

warned me how strange it is to have a baby and not keep it" (Peterson 1987, B4).

Who then are the surrogate mothers? Any fertile woman can volunteer to be a surrogate—the exact requisites depend on the country or on the agencies/clinics, and the anthropologist Helena Ragoné found that acceptance rates by agencies in the US ranged from 5 to 98% (Ragoné 1994, 26). The prospective surrogate mother is generally chosen because of her youth and good health status, and of her proven capacity to give birth. She normally has children of her own and often she must consider her family complete. Having children is generally required in order for her to evaluate the outcome of this experience on the basis of at least a previous one. But this rule is falsely reassuring, because first-time surrogates never had a child in order to give it away—though in fact some women did relinquish children for adoption, and they claim to want to revive the experience to feel in control when they depart from the child (Parker 1983). In India:

> The selection criteria for surrogates described by the commissioning parents, doctors, and agents in the course of the research [...] include physical attributes such as height and skin colour and other traits such as caste, religion, age, and children. Surrogates were also expected to be docile and not possess a *kadwa swabhav* (bitter/rude disposition). (Sama 2012, 25)

They must also have a husband who expresses his consent. Either intended parents choose the surrogate from a list, or mediators or clinics do it. Pande (2014, 138) found only one case of rejection of the couple by the surrogate. Interaction is minimal. Saroj was selected by the intended parents at a distance, then they traveled to meet her: "They came. They saw me. They left," she relates (Hochschild 2012, 80).

There is more space for negotiations in rich countries, where intended parents and surrogates meet personally, in the US after a match by agencies and in the UK during arranged meetings. In the US closed and open programs have a very different unfolding:

> In the closed programs, although couples select surrogates from a sheet of biographical data and a photograph provided by the programs, the surrogate does not have the same degree of choice about her couple, and the two parties do not interact with each other, meeting only to finalize the paternity suit and the step-parent adoption once the child is born. (Ragoné 1994, 14)

Nevertheless, "All programs advise couples and surrogates to terminate their relationship once the child is born, although photographs and cards for the holidays are considered appropriate in both open and closed programs" (Ragoné 1994, 18).

In the US nowadays there are many surrogates who do not want to "work" with third parties and select—and are selected by—the intended parents by announcements and personal knowledge. Knowing each other and meeting in person without intermediaries is also what the British model mandates by prohibiting advertisement.

The picture of this world from the '80s is rather bleak. The "first surrogate mother" delivered a baby in 1980 under the name of Elizabeth Kane. She was exhibited as a success story on the Phil Donahue Show and many other TV talk shows for more than a year. But when her son was six month old, she came to realize her family's and her own discomfort. A year later still, she broke ranks and voiced her sense of loss, joining the National Coalition Against Surrogacy[127] with the goal of banning commercial surrogacy because it exploited women:

> In January of 1985, I flew to England to speak out against surrogacy only weeks after the first British surrogate baby had been born. I told them we cannot ask women to have babies and give them away to men who are unhappy. That transferring one woman's pain to another person is not the solution in any society. (Kane 1989)[128]

Why had she wanted to do it then? As a Christian, she felt called to sacrifice herself, realizing only later that what she was asked for was inhumane, as she herself writes. She was used, felt merely a means to an end for the intended father, the "baby broker," and all the other promoters of surrogacy. She nevertheless had come to the idea of surrogacy herself:

---

[127] Still active as National Leadership Coalition Against Exploitation of Women by Use of Gestational Surrogacy Agreements, see their letter to Governor of New Jersey Christopher Christie on his Veto of Gestational Surrogacy, 31.7.2012 (http://www.cbc-network.org/wp-content/uploads/2012/08/NJ_Gov_Christie_Ltr_2012-08-08.pdf accessed 14.1.2015) and the Coalition Press Release on the Veto, 8 August 2012 (http://www.cbc-network.org/wp-content/uploads/2012/08/NJ_Press_Release_2012-08-08.pdf accessed 14.1.2015).

[128] She told her story in *Birth mother,* Harcourt, Brace, Jovanovich, 1988.

> My main motive at the time seemed to be altruistic. I had been surrounded by infertility all of my life [...] four or five of my friends were undergoing testing for infertility and our conversations revolved around trying to give their husband a child and their feelings of inadequacy at not being able to be a "good wife." We all knew it was our husband's job to supply material possessions and our job to take pride in our homes and to fill them with children. Those friends of mine who were Roman Catholic were expected to produce at least four or five children. Not only had they disappointed their husbands but their parents and the Pope. [...] As far back as 1970, I had talked to my husband about having a baby for a friend. I thought of it as an act of sisterhood.

The thought became serious in 1979:

> I read a UPI news article about an infertility specialist, Dr. Richard Levin, looking for a surrogate mother. I thought the name was quite appropriate since I would be substituting for another woman for nine months [...] I had convinced myself a scrawled signature on a contract would guarantee I would never love my child. I told myself daily during the entire pregnancy that this child was not mine, words frequently echoed by my baby broker. The fact that this couple already had an adopted son and were not childless did not bother me until I discovered it was the sperm donor who was obsessed with having a biological child. His wife was satisfied with the son they had adopted together.[129]
> I ached for her when she told me how empty she felt, knowing her husband had to hire a surrogate wife to prove his fertility. He had gained a child that had lived only in his imagination and I had lost a son who had been part of my life for eight and one half months.

The fact that the surrogacy was traditional gave her even more reason to regret it:

> I began receiving photographs of a beautiful brown eyed infant with chubby cheeks. He no longer looked exactly like his father as he did at the time of birth. Instead the top half of his face was identical to mine. Only then did I recognize the fact that he was MY SON, too. He would carry my genes with him from one generation into the next. And I had exchanged the right to never see him again for $11,500.
> I sank into a deep depression and had no interest in being a useful human being. I began to contemplate suicide as the only way to release my family from the shame they had suffered during my pregnancy. [...] My son did not ask to be deserted by me at birth. He did not decide he wanted to live in another state with a man I had never met.

---

[129] It seems that the choice of one or another kind of surrogacy is often made by "reconstructed families:" a new male partner comes to live with a woman that already has children and wants a child of his own, even if the woman is too old to conceive, or has become infertile after her last pregnancy. A US intended mother interviewed by the Swiss jurist Nora Bertschi finds, from her point of view, that men have a stronger will to reproduce (or rather, they do not bear the biological costs): "My boyfriend wasn't [infertile] and you know, for [a] man it's hard. [...] I wanted to give him his own child, it's hard to understand" (Bertschi 2014, 141).

The conclusion of Elizabeth Kane's speech is nevertheless positive: "My daughters will never play the martyr role my mother, my grandmother and I had been taught by our church and our society."

Phyllis Chesler interviewed 25 surrogate mothers, who all heard about this possibility from the Phil Donahue Show. The collective picture she gives is not a flattering one:

> the fanatical, almost stubborn naiveté exhibited by these women is almost impossible to convey. Happy or unhappy, they took great pride in how they trusted and obeyed everyone blindly about everything.
> These women believed whatever the surrogacy-clinic lawyers and doctors told them,. They rarely asked questions: they never disobeyed an order. They did exactly what they were told to do—and therefore couldn't "believe" that they'd been used for "one thing only," that they'd "never mattered," i.e., that their fantasies of being "above" it all had little to do with the realities of trafficking in women for profit. (Chesler 1988, 47)

And she adds:

> In a sense, a "good girl" *is*, by definition, a happy contract mother, that is, she is under reproductive contract either to her husband or to God himself. She is giving "the gift of life" to the unborn, to her husband, to a childless couple or to the world. (Chesler 1988, 48)

Anyway, some surrogates were critical of their own decisions. One found that having been an incest victim was her real motivation to act as a surrogate mother:

> Phyllis: (long pause) Would you say that deciding to be a "surrogate" is related to being an incest victim?
> Sally: Definitively. I hadn't reckoned how to cleanse my soul. How do I get my father's semen out of my body? I could accomplish this in the surrogate process. I could offer my body. This time, I was the one offering. Freely. This would somehow cleanse my soul.
> Phyllis: You thought being a surrogate would give you more control or retroactive control over your own body?
> Sally: Right. But it turned out to be totally wrong. The first insemination was the most horrible thing I ever went through in my whole life. It was like being an incest victim again! But I felt like I had to go through with it. Once I was pregnant, I couldn't have an abortion. I felt like I had to work this pregnancy through to heal myself. But what I did was to punish myself, not heal myself. (Chesler 1988, 66)

Another woman recalls that her support group for surrogate mothers did not support her at all when she started to have doubts about the feasibility of her promise. Another surrogate mothers' group in the UK would have certainly acted in this way also in the early '90s, as they created a subculture professionalizing surrogacy (Baslington 2002). But these problems could be attributed to the novelty of the practice. As for the case of Mary Beth Whitehead, the mother of Baby M, it can be argued that these dismaying episodes were just early cases, while nowadays there must be a self-selection of women who are apt to take the step of detachment.

The stances expressed in a Facebook group of people interested in surrogacy in Britain are indeed overwhelmingly positive: "I've been super priviledged to carry 3 surrogate babies for 3 different families been a joy and an honour" (accessed 10.12. 2014). An announcement in the internet to become a surrogate read: "I love being pregnant, although I am done having my own children. Being able to give the gift of a family to someone who can't have children is the most incredible feeling in the world." The gift of a new life elicits very positive comments: "Surrogacy is a beautiful thing" is the synthesis that many people make. These are the words of a grateful intended mother:

> The inability to have a family was earth shattering for myself and my partner, we had tried every route that ivf could offer us before we came across the amazing world of surrogacy and the wonderful ladies who have helped us. My first journey to have Myles and subsequent journeys have built friendships that are lifelong and unbelievably close to my heart. Pregnancy was as close to me carrying as possible, with attendance at all appintments, regular meet up with our surros and their lovely families, presence at the birth, and Myles was actually delivered into my arms. From that day till this, I have never struggled with any emotions other than pure love for my amazing son and our wonderful, giving surrogate. She is now part of the family, Myles's godmother and a dear friend and confident. The children, hers and ours, are happy confident children blessed to have a wonderful extended support network.

The language of "work" and its obligations is often present, though. In a presentation about surrogacy organized in Italy, a US surrogate said: "I wanted to work with them [the two intended parents], for me it is a way to build a bond with other people. It is one more thing in life that I wanted to experience." To a question about a possible change of heart, she answered: "I don't think you can agree to do something that has such a huge impact on other people and then walk away, I don't think you have the right to do it."[130] Still, being pregnant and giving birth has quite an impact on the woman herself, too.

---

[130] ELSA Taranto (the local branch of the European Law Students' Association) in collaboration with SISM Bari (Italian Secretary of Medicine Students), 17 April 2013 at "Dipartimento Jonico in Sistemi economici e giuridici del Mediterraneo: Società, Ambiente, Culture," Università degli Studi di Bari (http://www.youtube.com/watch?v=1uFvcAHxNlM accessed 1.9.2014).

The rewards for the surrogate mothers are the fulfilment of the values of self-sacrifice and of the altruistic mother's role taught to women, in front of a sympathetic audience constituted primarily of the intended parents. They feel good being able to donate the "ultimate gift," the gift of a new life:

> professing a love of children thus provides surrogates with an incontestable, socially acceptable motivation [...] she is performing an important task, helping an infertile couple to start a family of its own, an activity that, unlike an ordinary job, cannot be regarded as unfeminine, selfish, nonnurturant, or ambitious. (Ragoné 1994, 85 and 84)

Martha Field (1988, 20–21) relying mainly on press sources, lists among their disparate motives: the selfish experience of giving birth without having to care for the child, a private protest against abortion, the quest for the "perfect birth", and of course solidarity.

Former surrogates lead the non-profit agencies in the UK, extolling values like friendship and altruism (and acting as their gatekeepers to block researchers' requests for interviews, as the US forum moderators do).

In any case, the exceptionality of the situation is acknowledged: "No, I don't think everyone can do it. You have to be very, very strong" (Bertschi 2014, 137); "Not everyone can do it. It's like the steelworkers who walk on beams ten floors up: not everyone can do it, not everyone can be a surrogate" (Ragoné 1994, 85).

But regret about the relinquishment of one's baby is not a thing of the past, nor are the verdicts that separate birth mothers and children, even in countries where the birth mother's will should be respected according to the law. In 2009 an Australian court decided against a South African birth mother who had tried to get her baby back—the solemn prohibition of commercial surrogacy "down under" notwithstanding:

> *Rusken & Jenner* [2009] is the only published decision in which the foreign surrogate mother later resiled from her agreement to relinquish the child. That case principally concerned parenting orders that should be made as between the intended parents of the child, who were from South Africa and had entered into a surrogacy arrangement there. After the child was born, the intended parents moved to Australia with the child. The surrogate mother, who was from South Africa, intervened in the proceedings, seeking an order that the child should be returned to her in South Africa, on the basis of her right of custody over the child under South African law. Justice Bell emphasized that the surrogate mother was paid for her services, and rejected her claim that the child should be returned to her on the basis that there was no evidence that this would benefit the child. (Keyes 2013, 45)

But, as said, the cases of regret that go as far as disrupting the agreement and trying to keep or get the baby back, are rare.[131] Ragoné writes:

> with the exception of the Smith [fake name for a closed program] surrogates, none of the surrogates interviewed for this study expressed grief or sadness about parting with the baby (although they expressed sadness at the loss of the couple's attention and the surrogate role. (Ragoné 1994, 79)

The psychologist Bazel Baslington interviewed 14 British surrogates in 1992–3, a self-selected sample from a group of 430 surrogate mothers and infertile couples:

> According to their replies, the general experience was to feel unhappy in the short term but this passed fairly quickly. If a good relationship had been forged with the couple, this eased the relinquishment. Seven of the 14 mentioned the look on the faces of the couple as the baby is handed over to them as being "the best" part "… the expression of the parents' faces", or, "when they'd got the baby, you can't beat it". (Baslington 2002, 64–5)

In Hilary Hanafin's dissertation in 1984, "most of the surrogate mothers found comfort in knowing where the child was going and thought that this knowledge eased separation."[132] The conviction not to be pregnant for real, and in any case not with a baby who can be considered one's own is a shared feeling:

> I did this, knowing that it is not my baby and the embryo was created by them [the intended parents]. I was just the woman carrying it, so basically what I felt was a babysitter for nine months. […] I loved the baby, I care about her, but I have my own children. (Bertschi 2014, 143)

Social support to maintain this standpoint is essential. Open programs foster friendship between surrogate and intended parents: "It is the bond between

---

[131] The Oakland lawyer recounts: "In my time, I never had a surrogate who wanted to keep the child, never, ever. They like being pregnant. Intended parents find surrogates who have kids and are usually married. So they never...
Q: *When do they give up the baby?*
A: Right after birth. They don't usually breastfeed them. They pump their breast for several weeks and they get paid for that, until the 15th week or something like that. So they do never breastfeed them. And sometimes when they have children, who are younger, they often have young kids, and if they see mommy pregnant and everything, they say, can we have an hour with my kids, after birth, alone, in the room with my kids and the baby, and the parents are happy with that. They do that, sometimes, just because mommy is pregnant, there's a baby in there, and she has to explain that' (Personal interview, January 2013).

[132] Hilary Hanafin: *Surrogate mothers: an exploratory study*, Doctoral dissertation, California School of Professional Psychology, Los Angeles 1984 (reported by Baslington 2002, 59).

the couple and the surrogate, so carefully fostered by programs to substitute for the surrogate and child bond, that surrogates most often mourn" (Ragoné 1994, 44). The forum www.surromomonline.com has been followed by ZsuZsa Berend (2010) for more than six years: it works as a "collective consciousness" to summon "deviant" women to the shared values of the gift ethics, should a doubt arise about their role as containers for the "children" (i.e. fetuses) of others. In the following quote the role of the reminder of shared values was assumed directly by the intended mother:

> Gestational surrogates explain their lack of attachment by reference to both genetics and intent. One intended mother, who already had two children, reminded surrogates, "I am sorry that . . . you must experience pain and discomfort but please remember this isn't ALL about you. . . . You are having a miscarriage, yes, I realize that and it's miserable. . . . But please try to remember that it is my baby that died inside your body . . . life will be back to normal for you. I . . . will spend the rest of my life missing my unborn child. . . My arms will ache for the rest of my life to hold that baby."
> Her surrogate wholeheartedly agreed; this IM [intended mother] would "deserve that [baby] so much. . . . If there was another chance, I'd do it for you in a heartbeat!!" (Berend 2010, 252)

What the surrogate mothers feel when giving the children up is a mix of joy for the intended parents and pride for one's own performance: "It was just the best gift you could ever give anybody [...] giving them [the children] back was amazing [...] The look in their face, it's just beautiful [...] They just wanted it ever since" (Bertschi 2014, 145, interview with a US attorney).

An interesting observation by Kim Cotton regards the possible addictive nature of these feelings. She mentions it commenting the case of a surrogate who, despite getting older, is still proposing herself:

> What's driving her on is the delight she knows she can bring to these people. The problem with surrogates such as Jill is that I believe they become addicted to the "feel-good" factor of helping an infertile couple have a child. It is an absolutely amazing feeling. You are in a unique situation. You are the centre of this couple's world, you feel so special, and the bond you create with them—rather than the child—is what becomes so addictive. But unfortunately it doesn't last. Once the baby is born and the couple take their child away to start family life, it's over, even though they may stay in contact. This can be a very difficult time for the surrogate and the temptation for "just one more" is immense. (Weathers 2008)

Ragoné gives the context of these feelings: a working class background of surrogate mothers, who are enchanted by the opportunity to socially mix with professionals, while attesting to be satisfied with their primary maternal role:

> Surrogate programs take women whose lives revolve around their home and children or women who, when employed, view their employment as a financial necessity, a job rather than a career, and immerse them in an unfamiliar and interesting world filled with social interaction, beginning with the initial screening process, application forms, psychological evaluations, and physiological tests and continuing through a number of social interactions with professionals, couples, and other surrogates. From the moment she establishes the initial telephone contact with the program, a surrogate is made to feel important and special by the program staff. (Ragoné 1994, 63)

In other parts of the world the picture looks still bleak—from here. But on site in poor countries surrogacy represents a big economic opportunity for poor women and their families (or—sometimes, rather—the families they belong to).

Are they workers?

Even if at least some surrogate mothers in rich countries perceive and talk about what they are doing as work (though of a special and generous kind), they are never officially defined as workers even where contracts are legal. So the legal answer to the question of whether a surrogate mother is working is "no." But what the surrogate mother goes through has been labeled by critics of this practice as the ultimate expropriation of workers' products, the ultimate alienation. What if the birth mother is really just a worker who, like all the working class, is socially and legally forced to give away the product of her labor in the ultimate act of worker's alienation from the product of her efforts? Aren't pregnancy and delivery a part of the unpaid work that women perform to fulfill the social identity that a patriarchal and capitalist society has forced upon them in order to exploit their capacities, so that a rightful compensation should be claimed? In this case, the pregnancy work should not be any different if it is for one's own family or for another—though activists for wages for housework never endorsed producing babies for others as a job, nor singled out pregnancy in particular among the different socially reproductive activities of women for which a salary is due. Need surrogate mothers be looked upon as workers, and consequently the legal contract—as some authors have argued—be admitted to protect them?

The money to be gained is clearly the decisive factor for entering such an agreement in poor countries, or for poor people: "I have a girl who wants to start a shop in her village, another who wants to learn to cut hair and put up a beauty salon, another who wants to go to university," says a Mexican mediator, who employs women from Colombia.¹³³ But also in Europe migrant women find work as surrogates. A Bolivian woman relates:

> "I came to Spain because I couldn't find work in my country. But even here I can't earn enough money to send back to support my family. I want to become a surrogate mother so I can return quicker to my home with enough money to look after my daughter." She plans to meet prospective couples in Spain before travelling back to Bolivia with them for impregnation at a private clinic as such practices are forbidden under Spain's Assisted Reproduction law. She will then stay in her country and give birth to the baby. (Govan 2006)

In Israel surrogacy is openly a job:

> The Israeli surrogates in my study shared many of the same stated motivations as US and British surrogates, such as love of pregnancy, empathy for childless couples, and the desire to make a unique contribution, but they were also unapologetic, honest, and upfront about money being their primary goal in pursuing surrogacy. They expressed diverse economic goals that ranged from the immediate, such as paying off huge debts and providing for their children's basic needs, to the less immediate, such as saving money for the future. (Teman 2010, 23)

The job is taken up enthusiastically by many for its altruistic (or self-sacrificing) side and because it involves babies and family building. One of the Columbians recalls: "Since when I was a kid I played with dolls—children fascinate me, they enchant me, I adore them. If there is a couple or a family who needs a baby to be happy, and you make them perfectly happy, I want to contribute." Another says: "I can contribute to somebody else's happiness, and make a new experience."

Many women are not only economically but also psychologically coerced into something they do not really give an informed consent to, as they are not either explained or talked to directly, but accept what their family tells them to do. The anthropologist Amrita Pande did an ethnography in India with 52 pregnant surrogate mothers for nine months in the clinic and hostel where they lived. She found that the group was basically divided into three: those who were taking independent decisions, not only to enter a surrogacy agreement, but also in many other areas of their lives, and controlled their earnings;¹³⁴ those who were persuaded (not completely…) by a broker;

---

[133] Journeyman TV (https://www.youtube.com/watch?v=4SYBxY2NHaQ accessed 15.10.2014).

[134] One of them says: "Women have to bear so much of sadness for this, why should they give the money to their husbands? And in any case what does he have to do in this? He did nothing. At least the other man gave his sperm, not that that is a very big task either" (Pande 2014, 152).

those who were not able to make decisions, even on their pregnancies, as these decisions were taken by their husbands and families instead. All medical decisions were taken by intended parents. Sama, a Delhi-based group working in women's and health issues, denounces what happens normally:

> The "patients" that the doctors were catering to were the commissioning parents, and not the surrogates. The surrogate's identity was reduced to the pages kept in a file and was largely perceived as an appendage to the commissioning parents. She was regarded as someone who would otherwise not have been able to access the services of the medical establishment, and was treated in a decidedly inferior manner. [...] This was evident in her assuming that the doctors or the staff would not welcome any communication from her, especially her asking them questions. The medical ethical protocols of securing the surrogate's consent were meant to be followed in this forbidding and alien setting. This raises serious doubts about the possibility of gaining consent in a free and equitable manner, given the hindrances and disadvantages faced by surrogates. (Sama 2012, 76–77)

A concrete example from their interviews:

> *They had transferred four eggs (embryos) inside me and I was not told about it. One day, I got a call asking me to visit the hospital. They told me that one of the children did not have a heartbeat and that one has to be taken out by surgery. I was very scared. I didn't understand how you could take one out. What if something happens to me? I called my husband, but before he could reach, they had taken me inside for the surgery. That night there was too much pain in my stomach. (SD6)...*
> Since it was the commissioning parents who were considered the "patients" in the case of surrogate pregnancies, the question of acquiring the surrogate's consent was bypassed or ignored time and again, and information was shared only with the commissioning parents. (Sama 2012, 66)

Even communication with other surrogates is forbidden:

> *You can get into trouble if you ask too much. The most you can ask is where are you from. Asking more than that can get you into trouble.* (Sama 2012, 78)

The highly medicalized management of the surrogate pregnancies means an increased burden on the health of the birth mothers:

> Furthermore, the injections and pills used to prevent lactation have serious side effects, ranging from dizziness and nausea to hair loss, etc. There is also the possibility of breast engorgement, an extremely painful condition, which may arise if the woman who is lactating is not allowed to breast feed. (Sama 2012, 70)

Also a commentator from Russia protests current medical treatments:

> This raises serious questions about the kinds of procedures that qualify as "medically indicated" and why the successful birth and the delivering of the child to the commissioning parents should be achieved at the cost of the surrogate's health. (Rivkin-Fish 2013, 83)

A woman interviewed by Pande recounts a crime of forced abortion (here the synthesis by Hochschild):

> Parvati, a thirty-six-year-old Akanksha surrogate, learned, after the fact, that in signing her contract (which was written in English) she had signed over the right to decide whether or not to abort a baby. At Akanksha, surrogates were usually implanted with many eggs, and when three or more survived, Dr. Patel routinely aborted the "extras." When Parvati found she was pregnant with triplets, Dr. Patel told her that one had to go. Distressed, she told Amrita Pande 'I'll keep one, After all, it's my blood even if it's their genes'[135] [...] Against Parvati's wish, Dr. Patel aborted one fetus. (Hochschild 2012, 98)

Pande finds that the surrogates she lived with during her fieldwork did not know much about the medical procedures, and had little control over the payments. They adored Doctor Madam, the founder of the clinic, to whom they were grateful for that economic opportunity. Her disciplinary project was to make them the perfect surrogate: "Cheap, docile, selfless and nurturing;" "To be a perfect surrogate, a woman has to be a good mother first and then a good contract worker" in delivering the baby (Pande 2014, 64 and 74). To be sure of this, the women in labor are made to undergo a C-section, and when they wake up from the anesthesia the baby is normally gone. Surrogates rarely can breast-feed. Nevertheless, differently from Israel where surrogates exercise mental control to detach themselves from their pregnancy, Indian surrogate mothers testify a continuing sense of belonging with their contract children: "She is my first baby girl. I have two sons and I always craved for a girl. I know she looks Japanese, but I think of her as my own daughter" (Pande 2014, 149). In Hochschild's interview with an infertile couple from the US looking for an Indian surrogate, their ignorance about the situation they stepped into is highlighted:

---

[135] Original source: "She opposed the fetal reduction surgery that eliminated one of the fetuses she carried: 'Madam told us that the babies won't get enough space to move around and grow, so we should get the surgery. But Nandinididi [the intended mother] and I wanted to keep all three. I told Doctor Madam that I'll keep one and Nandinididi can keep two. We had informally decided on that. After all it's my blood even if it's their genes. And who knows whether at my age I'll be able to have more babies'" (Pande 2010, 308).

> Although Tim and Lili were able to imagine the poverty of Indian surrogates, they had no sense of the emotional challenges they faced, especially that of retaining their dignity. Tellingly, dormitory gossip among the surrogates targeted those who were "too practical" about their job. Amrita Pande found, for example, that Anjali was roundly criticized by the other surrogates who felt that she had become too driven, too strategic, and too materialistic. She had her fancy new house, her children in private schools, her stereo, her DVDs, and she still wanted more. They all needed money and they were all renting their wombs to earn it. But as a matter of dignity, the surrogates felt there were limits, their bodies were not just moneymaking machines. Granted, there was little talk among them of surrogacy as an act of altruism, and many admitted enjoying aspects of their nine months of dormitory life. "Ice cream, coconut water, and milk, every day—and they are paying for it!" one surrogate told Pande [2014, 152], adding; "I think I deserve it for all I am doing right now."
> Nonetheless, they drew a firm line. Yes, they had babies for money, but they strongly resisted the idea that materialism had suppressed their motherly feelings. As one put it, "We will remember our babies all of our lives." So, some surrogates condemned Anjali for carrying babies only for money, and for being therefore "like a whore"—a dishonor they all feared. Poignantly, even surrogates desperate for money took pride in not becoming *too* money-minded, and in feeling that they were giving the gift of life. (Hochschild 2012, 94–5, cf. Pande 2014, 160 ff.)

But the work of Pande in fact shows how the worker is "produced" by disciplinary practices in order to obtain a mother-worker, who takes motherly care of the content of her womb while pregnant, but acts with the detachment of a worker when the baby is ready to be extracted.

An Indian gynecologist considers: "Only someone who is in desperate need for money will do surrogacy, otherwise carrying someone else's baby for nine month is not something which is really acceptable. So only someone who is really desperate comes [...] to surrogacy" (Bertschi 2014, 193). Pande agrees: "Surrogacy is undertaken as a sense of familial duty, out of economic desperation and not as an occupation of choice" (Pande 2014, 132).

Cheap Indian surrogates are sought after not only from rich countries (successful Indian migrants included), but also by wealthy couples from Sri Lanka, Pakistan, Nepal, Bangladesh, Thailand, and Singapore (Smerdon 2008, 23). Surrogacy often comes after the experience of egg "donation" at a clinic, where it is proposed to be able to participate in surrogacy. It is an investment, as the broker must immediately be paid 200 USD:

> The story is oft repeated in Anand. To begin with, women donate their eggs—usually for Rs. 5000 [81 USD]—and then go on to renting their wombs. A successful surrogacy could mean anything from Rs. 1.5 lakh to Rs. 3 lakhs [2,400–4,800 USD]—many times more than their annual household income. (Ghosh 2006)

In this poor and highly unequal country, the money earned does make a difference in the lives of surrogates (though, sadly, not for a long time, as Pande recounts in her last chapter):

> But I have done this because of my poverty. Otherwise I would never have taken this step.
> At that time I was suffering from lot of financial problems and my husband told me I can sell my kidney to pay the debt, but I said, no need, I will do surrogacy. (Documentary *Made in India* 2010)

In Israel the same tragic alternative was related for the most destitute group of surrogates: "They sometimes mentioned that surrogacy was a better option for resolving their situation than other options they had considered, such as selling a kidney" (Teman 2010, 24).

Nevertheless, even in these extreme (and blatantly unethical, as true consent cannot be established because of withheld information) situations, these women perceive their "gift of life" as something that cannot really be bought, as is shown by the ethnographic work of Kalindi Vora on an Indian clinic she calls Manushi:

> Many of the surrogate mothers I spoke to, all of whom were Hindu or Christian, emphasized a feeling that they were doing something great, often in the religious language of being like a god, or being able to give a gift to an infertile couple that is a gift usually given only by God. Most were usually quick to then include the doctors as part of this ability to provide, but the emphasis was on their own power to give. Those who spoke to this topic emphasized that this exalted aspect of their actions was much more important than the money aspect, and in fact was their primary motivation. (Vora 2010–11, 4)

Pande instead finds that for the surrogates she followed, the rhetoric of "the gift of life" does not make sense: "How can a desperately poor woman from a village in India possibly be giving a gift to an upper-class Caucasian couple from Los Angeles?" (Pande 2014, 92). She also finds that the "divine" was rather an attribute for the opportunity they received to raise their family out of poverty (however temporarily). Plus, Doctor Madam's deeds were divine. Both Vora and Pande attribute these expressions to indoctrination by the clinic:

> In discussing the anticipation of parting with the infant upon its birth, a number of the women working as surrogates explained independently that since the baby wouldn't look like her, she wouldn't feel a bond with it. This explanation is used by doctors to guide surrogates in thinking of the child as not their own. Despite this coaching and the understanding that the babies are not theirs, women who had already delivered did say they missed the infants after they left India and hoped to hear about their development, receive pictures of the children, and maintain a connection to these families. (Vora 2010–11, 3)

The analogy between the land and the womb strikes Vora, too:

> For example, the re-formulation of the surrogates' bodies as empty spaces that can be cultivated to re-produce Western society and Western lives recapitulates the colonial epistemology of land as property, where resources, including native labor, were used to sustain the metropole. (Vora 2010–11, 5)

Not only at the material, but also at the symbolic level, expropriation is pervasive. Vora describes in this way her interactions at the Manushi clinic:

> The surrogates I spoke to, including former and current surrogates and women full of hope waiting to find out whether they had become pregnant as surrogates, first described surrogacy to me in the manner they assumed I wanted to hear, as it was what clinic staff, doctors, and former surrogates counselled them to understand and accept: the uterus is a space in a woman's body that is empty when she is not expecting a child, and surrogacy is simply the renting out of that space for someone else's child. (Vora 2013)

> The lack of a genetic link made possible through IVF technology is presented to surrogates as evidence of the lack of biological connection to the child, and thus as grounds for surrogates having no claim on the child. The proposed legislation to regulate surrogacy in India also clearly states that the surrogate has to relinquish all her rights over the child. (Sama 2012, 64)

Interview excerpts from Indian surrogates are distressing. Not only is a surrogate made to believe that she is not the mother, but sometimes even that this pregnancy is different:

> I was only explained this thing, that once I begin taking my medicine and I have the embryo transfer, something like a bubble, like we have the water bubbles […] would be placed in my womb with the help of medicine and doctors intervention and that slowly, slowly will begin growing for nine month and then you give that to the parents. (Bertschi 2014, 187)

This representation is coherent with the patriarchal vision of procreation in ART times: "Politically and legally, technological reproduction tends to position the fetus as isolated and independent from the mother but not from the sperm source, the doctor, or the state" (Raymond 1994, xii). Of course if women embrace patriarchy, it is easier for them:

> This cultural tendency to trivialize gestation and to privilege genetic determinism perhaps eliminated certain conflicts between the Israeli surrogates and intended mothers I studied; by way of comparison, when gestational influence is believed to be highly consequential to fetal outcome, conflict may erupt, for example, over the surrogate's nutrition during pregnancy. (Teman 2010, 61)

As in India it is socially unacceptable to be pregnant with somebody else's baby, the women either hide their pregnancy or hide themselves, living at the clinics' dorms. This is also convenient to keep them under surveillance, lest they harm the fetus. This is how some surrogates were kept in a world-famous clinic (Pande's field notes from 2006):

> The room is lined with eight beds, one next to the other with barely enough space to walk in between. A ceiling fan groans above, some of the beds are raised on one side with a block so that the women can have their legs elevated after the embryo transfer or any gynecological checkups. There is nothing else in the room. Each bed has a pregnant woman resting on it. This is their home for the next few months. Their husbands can visit, but not stay the night. It's a reminder that they cannot have sex. Not for the next few months. The women are still in their nightclothes, and it's nearly evening. The day has been planned for them, the morning visit from the doctor, 8 am breakfast, 9 am medicines, 10 am rest hour, 12 pm injections, followed by an afternoon nap. The evening is nothing different. Except perhaps the broker will bring in a new member. A bed will be added to the room. Another pregnant woman will join the ranks. (Pande 2014, 2)

But Pande warns the reader that in India surveillance and disciplining of workers is much the same in other sectors, if not worse. Also the surrogates quite enjoy their stay, a long break from their daily drudgery:

> Of course, I don't like not being able to go home to my children. But I also don't mind staying here. Right now my son takes care of all the housework. But once I go back I will go back to being a mother, a house cleaner, a farmer; everything again! And it's not like I just work at home, I also clean other people's houses. All this [pampering—note by Pande] is my way of getting something back. Do you know, I sometimes ask my husband to give me a foot massage. I am sure he doesn't like that! (Pande 2014, 123)

And confined surrogates create their own social relationships based on affection and solidarity, subverting their socially assigned role:

> They disrupt the construction of Indian kinship as a bounded sphere constrained by not just patriliny but also interactions within the same caste and religion. For daily existence and negotiations, shared company, continuous labor and the effort of reciprocities take precedence over formal and restrictive models of interactions, and ties of "sisterhood" seemingly cross all borders. (Pande 2014, 164)

Nevertheless, she continues, "The everyday and creative kin ties established by the surrogates may pose very little threat to the fundamental (genetic) foundation of kinship." And, for what concerns international ties, the policy of the clinics is normally of not allowing contact between surrogates and intended parents before and during the pregnancy, and most certainly not afterwards. The surrogates with whom Pande lived were hurt by this attitude. Often the intended parents' interest is just feigned:

> Munni seems surprised by the sudden severing of ties. Her relationship with her clients was unusually friendly while she was carrying their baby. But once she completed her contract, her reproduction became a classic example of alienated labor. Her clients honored the capitalist contract: they paid her and appropriated the surplus value of her reproductive labor—the baby. (Pande 2014, 184)

Or their interest is misdirected:

> While some intended parents write to their surrogates and send email correspondence and photos of the infant in the first year, most of the surrogates said they do not hear from their former clients very frequently. The clients I spoke to tended to express a feeling of connection to "India" rather than to individual women, some mentioning that they would inform their children of the circumstances of their birth or that they hoped to bring the child to India someday to see where it was born, but not necessarily to visit the clinic or surrogate. (Vora 2010–11, 2)

Let us go back to a country with rule of law and of contract. My Californian interviewees were very happy about the enforceability of the agreement because it made everybody's position clear:

> I think everybody thinks it's the reasonable thing to do, once you have consenting adults entering into a contract, an arrangement, that then they should be able to be bound by it, which is the big issue.
> *Question: What is the most difficult part? To find the surrogate?*
> Answer: Finding the surrogates is not so easy, we try to recruit some surrogates through the clinic here, but it's not so easy. It's not an easy thing to do, medically maybe it's the easiest thing to do, but other things are not so easy, so I think the medical part is not difficult, but all negotiations about the legal things to do and dealing with the pregnancy and the complications or what if the surrogate is to be bedrest and cannot work, these all kinds of things that must be worked in the contract. […] I think most of the times surrogates are to be women who are stable, that enjoy being pregnant,[136] that have a stable situation preferably and that are not so desperate for money they would do anything… and so you want to find a situation where you have the smallest number of risks. If you just make an ad and put it out that you are gonna pay 25,000 dollars to car-

---

[136] This is a set phrase of the surrogates, exposed by Ragoné: "Based on the data gathered in this study, it can be concluded that it is not the ease of pregnancy that informs a surrogate's decision to become a surrogate; neither is it, as surrogates often state, that they 'enjoy being pregnant' or that 'pregnancy is a breeze,' although for some this may be true. It is clear that surrogates have experienced miscarriages and ectopic pregnancies, have had difficulty conceiving, and have been given infertility drugs, synthetic hormones to expedite conception, and that none of these obstacles discourage or dissuade surrogates" (Ragoné 1994, 62).

ry out a pregnancy for you, you are going to get a lot of responses, but most of these people you don't wanna work with and it's hard for parents who desperately want to have children, to reject someone who says they're gonna help them. (Personal interview with gynecologist, January 2013)

Generosity notwithstanding, the term "work" is often employed to describe the task of the surrogate in rich countries, too. The doctor speaking habitually used the verb "to work" for the surrogate, e.g.: "We occasionally have some surrogates who work without an agency." Announcements over the internet read: "I do not work with agencies"—which can also in fact mean that to be involved with an agency would transform what the woman is doing into work. But other contexts clarify that in the US the verb is properly employed:

> Psychologists at the monthly meetings repeatedly encouraged surrogates to refer to each other as "colleagues" and to think of themselves as "professionals." This deliberate professionalization of the surrogacy experience makes it difficult for surrogates to share honestly about personal doubts they may have about the choice they've made, the center's practices, or the couple they "work" for, because they would seem unprofessional. (Ragoné 1996, 354)

More or less in the same period the same was happening in the UK: "I discovered that the surrogate mother members were *encouraged* by the self help group to think of their surrogacy arrangement as a job incorporating payment" (Baslington 2002, 58). With Zelizer, this mix of money and intimacy shouldn't be considered a moral problem for gestational services either, and in fact moral boundaries (shifting with lowered standards following material need) are re-traced by surrogate mothers in order not to consider themselves as "baby-sellers:"

> I think they [the intended parents] chose us because of Shalin [Divya's infant son]. He was very healthy then. They liked him so much that they wanted just to take him home with them! But we were sure about one thing, no one and nothing can make us give away our own child. *We are not like that. We won't sell our baby.* (Pande 2014, 132)

But the foundations of these fine cultural distinctions, affirming that the truly unacceptable act would be to sell "one's own" babies (i.e. those not conceived for that purpose), seem shaky. Differently from India, in rich countries surrogacy is not considered by participants as selling anything. But in the context of compensation or reimbursement, just how long does it take a surrogate to shift gear from generous helping to baby-selling? The British surrogates interviewed by Hazel Baslington belonged to a subculture that valued payment for surrogacy: "I am paid to do a job, to keep the emotions a little at bay" (Baslington 2002, 64). This seems to reveal a paradoxical situation: altruistic surrogacy is possible only if it is paid for.

The reading of the self-help guide from one surrogate to her "colleagues" again reveals the effort to be professional: "A Gestational Surrogate is a woman who carries and has no biological relationship to the children she is carrying. PERIOD" (Alexander 2006, 3). Her booklet mainly contains advice on how to be professional and not be cheated economically, but rightfully compensated for all the procedures undergone, either successful or not:

> "Canceled cycle"
> You have completed your med protocol for the transfer and it is time for the transfer. Something goes terribly wrong—your cycle is canceled. What are the circumstances surrounding the canceled cycle? The reason for cancellation could range from surrogate lining issues to ED [egg donation] issues. There have been many cases where surrogates get to days before the transfer and their body just stops cooperating. It hurts. Hurts to know that after all you have done to get this far, your body does otherwise.
> Let us just say, it was not as a result of your body. Did you add a canceled cycle fee in your contract? If not, and you are reading this book prior to completion of your contract—hurry up and write it down. A lot of surrogates that have had canceled cycles and failed to include this stipulation in the contract tend to kick themselves in the behind later. Remember—always put yourself and your family first. (Alexander 2006, 54).

In exchange for this professionalism, Alexander encourages them not to sign "all-inclusive" contracts, but to break down all the expenses, not accepting caps on any item of the list:

> Base fee
> Multiple fee
> Monthly expense allowance
> Maternity clothing allowance
> Transfer fee
> Mock cycle fee
> Dropped/canceled cycle fee
> Invasive procedure fee
> C-section
> Life insurance
> Housekeeping fee
> Baby-sitting fee
> Travel
> Medical coverage
> Legal expenses (Alexander 2006, 41)

As Alexander puts it, in fact, women do surrogacy for the advantage of their own families. This can be easily translated as "for the money they get"—as their families hardly get any other benefits out of it. On the contrary, it is often observed that the other children of the surrogate fear that they will be removed from the family, too.

Goslinga-Roy describes the motivation of the surrogate mother in her ethnography in the US:

> The fee was also insufficient to compensate for the sacrifices—this was a term Julie used—both she and her husband would have to make, which she felt were "not about money." For example, the daily regimen of hormone injections the first two months of the pregnancy left her buttocks looking like pin-pricked cushions for months; she and her husband would have to abstain from sexual relations for the duration of the pregnancy; frequent appointments with physicians and phone calls to Pamela Martin, the child's ultimate mother, ate into her time with her family; she would be giving birth, risking physical harm and even death; and she would most likely endure engorged breasts again as she had with her own son. When I asked midway through the pregnancy why she was not growing resentful about these impositions on her body, her person, her family, and her time—they seemed overwhelming to me—she replied that it wouldn't make sense to most people, but these "sacrifices" were in fact fine with her. (Goslinga-Roy 2000, 119–120)

The theme of self-sacrifice is paramount in narrations of surrogates. For example in this self-presentation of a woman willing to act as a surrogate in a Facebook group she mentions future contact as legitimized (also) by further sacrifices on her part:

> Im N. im 23 I wasnt to be a TS surrogate. I have 2 boys
> As a sorragate Id like pictures and updates from time to time and depending on what we agreed to meet up a couple of times a year. Obviously the child will eventually want to know and im ok with that and it's up to parents what happens with that Even if no contact id like updates yearly at minimum on how they are doing. If they got really majorly sick id like to be informed. .if they needed a kidney etc as obv I may be a match
> The reason i want to do it is I had endometriosis and was told I couldn't have babies...I had 2 and it calmed my endometriosis right down and I was devestated when I thought I couldn't so I want to help others and it helps me at the same time with when I do get pain as when pregnant it stops any pain and helps it get better

Christian beliefs, as for Elizabeth Kane, explain this attitude, despite the general contrariness of churches. In Hilary Hanafin's dissertation two thirds of the studied group were "traditional" or "conservative" women, while Helena Ragoné only found 5%—that equals just one nontraditional surrogate out of 28 interviewed.[137] Zsuzsa Berend found religious attitudes, too:

---

[137] Hilary Hanafin: *Surrogate mothers: an exploratory study*, Doctoral dissertation, California School of Professional Psychology, Los Angeles 1984 (quoted by Ragoné 1994, 56).

> Surrogates also often assert that "God is the only creator of life. I also believe He's all knowing. So, God knows what's going on and if He wants this life to be created through surrogacy then He's not creating a baby for me, He's creating it for my IPs. Therefore, I'm not giving up my baby. I'm simply handing over theirs" (Berend 2010, 251–252)

In Thailand, besides money, self-sacrifice and religion are both powerful motivators: "Several women used the term *tan-bun* (merit-making) to explain their motivation to become a surrogate. *Tan-bun* is a term that means a meritorious and good act" (Hibino and Shimazono 2013, 64). But in the US it is surrogacy itself that is worth dying for: "I had a rough delivery, a C-section, and my lung collapsed because I had the flu, but it was worth every minute of it. If I were to die from childbirth, that's the best way to die. You died for a cause, a good one" (Ragoné 1994, 82).

Feminist authors (e.g. Raymond 1990 and 1994, Folbre 2001, Federici 2012) have correctly indicated how self-sacrifice is constitutive of female identity also in contemporary capitalism and how women's unpaid work underpins the money sector: "We have to make clear that, within the wage, domestic work produces not merely use values, but is essential to the production of surplus value" (Dalla Costa and James 1972, 9). And it is true, as Raymond emblematically describes, that the costs to the birth mother are huge, and that this reverberates on the social position of women:

> Women give their bodies over to painful and invasive IVF treatments when it is often their husbands who are infertile. Women are encouraged to offer their bodies in a myriad of ways so that others may have babies, health, and life. These noble-calling and gift-giving arguments reinforce women as self-sacrificing and ontological donors of wombs and what issues from them. Altruistic reproductive exchanges leave intact the status of women as a breeder class. Women's bodies are still the raw material for other's needs, desires, and purposes. (Raymond 1990, 11)

Raymond also correctly points out that not only the market is a site of exploitation, but the family, too: "The potential for women's exploitation is not necessarily less because no money is involved and reproductive arrangements may take place within a family setting" (Raymond 1990, 9).

Should we thus dismiss the birth mothers' conviction that they are acting out of benevolence, that they are not workers, only by looking at the "big picture," the general usefulness of a numerous population for capitalist development included? No, the levels are two and must not be confused. We cannot substitute the subjects' interpretation of their actions for the observers' interpretation, as the two belong to different levels of analysis: the culture in and about surrogacy on one hand, and on the other the observers' (as objective as possible) analysis of what is going on from the material point of view. If there are newborns on one hand and money on the other and the two get punctually exchanged, this is objectively called buying and selling. If no money changes hands, the subjective experience of having done a good and generous deed is confirmed by the observations. Plus, the individual paid good deed quickly becomes a social obligation. On the internet birth mothers who want to keep their babies are ferociously condemned in forums and comments spaces. These are some reactions, following the case of a woman carrying twins for her gay brother and his husband (she also appears in *Breeders*). Their relationship deteriorated, ending in a long litigation. The article commented on, written by Ted Sherman (2011), reports both the judge's decision (noting the likely damage of the "strong feelings about homosexuality and surrogacy" harbored by the birth mother) and her attorney's denial of the relevance of the father's sexual orientation to the birth mother's actions. These are some of the comments:[138]

> Comment: christineATtheyknownot Dec 20, 2011
> I think giving her visitation is wrong unless it was in the surrogacy document. This isn't hard to figure out.
> A: The couple wanted children.
> B: The couple found a willing surrogate.
> C: The surrogate had the children.
> D: The surrogate decided that she wanted the children.
> E: The surrogate sues.
> The surrogate is not in any way biologically related. The surrogate was on contract to give the children to the couple. She has NO rights. None. Zip. Zilch. Zero.
> This court giving her visitation is too much.
> If she wants to see the kids, she needs to kiss up to her brother and his husband.
> This is a case of parent rights. She is not the parent. Biologically and legally *HE* is.
> NJvotr64 Dec 21, 2011 @Christine
> I completely agree with you. I don't see that she should have any legal visitation rights and I'm surprised the judge did that. Do surrogates usually get legal visitation rights? She isn't even the biological mother. She is the babies' aunt and if the family can settle their issues than she can see them as their aunt.
> They wanted a baby and she agreed to carry their baby, knowing they were gay. Quite frankly, she shouldn't get any say in how these babies are raised!!!

---

[138] Posted in http://www.nj.com/news/index.ssf/2011/12/nj_gay_couple_fight_for_custod.html accessed 10.9.2014.

> Mary Lee Greer Dec 20, 2011
> I'm sorry, did this woman think she was going to get paid to get a baby? I've offered to be a surrogate to someone close to me who can't have children and at no point in time have I ever thought that I would be considered the child's mother. Of course I would want to be involved in the child's life, but as an aunt, not as a parent. I need to look up the Mary Beth Whitehead case, because unless the parents who hired the surrogate backed out, I don't see why the surrogate would be the mother.
>
> ll4mmep Dec 20, 2011
> I see why the judge gave the twins to Sean because it was his actual sperm that was used with a donor egg. Ok. Angelia's only ties to the twins is that she carried them.
> 1 post on the attachment, if she does not have other kids
> Pregnancy is not only a physical transition, it is also mental and when women agree to go through with this process all things need to be considered before agreeing. nicky823
>
> pebbles07 I am seriously disgusted that this woman, the man's sister nonetheless!, felt that she could dictate how to raise the children and fight these men for custody. They are obviously in a committed, loving relationship. She knew that they were homosexual before agreeing to carry the children. And now she wants to act like she's "mom" because she carried the children for 10 months. Pathetic.

Only in the second half of the comments we can find an opinion more or less sympathetic with the birth mother:

> ammon44 Dec 20, 2011
> Any woman who has a child finds it nearly impossible to give the baby up if she holds it and spends time with it. That is just instincts and human nature. Adoption agencies have found that if the mother holds the baby for any length of time the adoption will be called off so they try to encourage the mother to give the baby up as soon as possible. The mistake they made, among many, was having his sister do it and then letting her be around her babies. Those maternal instincts are very strong. I doubt it was so much about the homosexual issue as it was about wanting her babies. Stop judging the poor woman as a bigot and realize she carried those babies for 9 months and then gave birth to them, which is an act of love where the mother literally risks her life for them. It is understandable that any woman would want to keep them after going through that, contract or no contract.

This deviant voice is immediately rebuffed:

> JRZINTEGRITYNOW Dec 20, 2011
> Her only instinct is for self-preservation. I'd love to see why she had a life-threatening birth . . .drugs maybe . . .why was she "dependent" on her brother and couldn't use her own eggs??? I have a sister like that. . . I wouldn't want one of her eggs and wouldn't even use her as a "vessel" to have my baby no matter how desperate I was. There's more to this that's not being told.

It is astonishing how even gay men—provided that they are married and want to reproduce—can elicit more sympathy on the web than a woman who has become a mother. She must be really bad.

Bad women

In the first publicly debated cases of surrogacy, the US birth mother, Mary Beth Whitehead, and the pregnant English woman, Kim Cotton, were both depicted in the media as avid and selfish. Kim Cotton—who has always defended surrogacy and later organized it as a founding member of the association COTS—found herself morally condemned for what she thought of as a generous choice (in fact she was paid much more by the media for exclusive interviews than the amount she received from the intermediating agency: 15,000 GBP compared to 6,500). It is ironic that neither the good deeds of the surrogates nor the "win-win" situation of their exchanges with the intended parents[139] are acknowledged by many commentators, who would rather compare surrogate mothers to whores, generally advocating for a prohibition of surrogacy just as prostitution is forbidden in many states (for example in nearly all the US, and in many ex-colonies by legacy of European prohibitionist penal codes). Andrea Dworkin in fact called the surrogates "the new prostitutes" (1983, 181–188) and Kajsa Ekis Ekman (2013) encompasses the two situations in her abolitionist battle to save female victims of both social institutions. The parallel is obvious: the use of women's sexual parts is exchanged for money (though also men and transgenders work in prostitution), while third parties are pushing them to enter the agreements in order to get a share of their gains.[140] These acts, according to abolitionist feminists, must be forbidden and fought against, culturally and legally. Traditionalist arguments also equate prostitution and commercial surrogacy. Public condemnation threatens women who are (or seem to be) coldly calculating their own material interest in areas where they are supposed to be subservient, generous and selfless: love/sex relationships and motherhood. This is sometimes expressed in the form of women's loss of dignity—but traditional morality unswervingly abhors both the heartless mothers who abandon their children and the whores. In fact, gut reactions invoking prohibitions for particular acts of disposal of women's sexual capacities often mask

---

[139] Even in India: "the 'surrogacy industry' constructs the discourse of a win-win scenario for both infertile couples and women struggling with poverty. On both the demand and supply sides, one notices the emergence of a society in which individuals do not depend on the state for any solutions," comments an Indian feminist group (Sama 2012, 25).

[140] It can also be the very same women: "Surrogacy services now available in Nigeria" http://nigerianescorts.blogspot.it/2013/10/surrogacy-services-now-available-in_1.html accessed 3.1.2015.

the age old fear that women lose their generosity, femininity, attitude to care, to become a *mulier œconomica*, the feminine counterpart of the selfish subject that social theories originating in the 19th century still postulate (Folbre 2009). It is understood that if women lose their giving "nature," the non-capitalist basis of capitalist society would crumble and fall (Dunaway 2014). One of the paradoxes of capitalism is that its monetary sphere "rests" on a base of unpaid work—to use the Braudelian metaphor visualising economic relations as a three-storey building: on a vast base of "daily life" an upper floor of competitive markets elevates itself, topped by a dominating and monopolistic floor of capitalism. The capitalist circuit of profit would immediately be blocked, should social reproduction be paid for. "Love," generous and free, is the cliché that is supposed to motivate the only approved use of women's capacities (also sexual). In the case of prostitution, the harsh judgment on women practicing it, is in fact an ancestral stigma imposed on "loose women," those who do not use their sexuality in the modest, or non-existent, way prescribed, and in so doing worsen their social position (generally already low, unless they consort with powerful men). It is the typical case of double morality: men are always appreciated better the more sexual partners they have, while the "whore stigma" hangs like a Damocles' sword over all females, regardless if they are paid for sex or if they enjoy it (sometimes both happen).

But, besides the double morality, there are other arguments against prostitution. Abolitionist feminists have come to the conclusion that it is not possible to consider sex work as a job because women who accept money to perform sexual acts submit themselves to sexual violence even if they superficially consent to it. Intimate acts lose their meaning and sex is forced upon them, provoking serious mental problems such as post-traumatic stress syndrome (not true: see Vanwesenbeek 1994, still the only reliable psychological research on sex workers and a control group). But prostitution is only a part of a much broader sexual-economic exchange between the sexes, that Paola Tabet (1998) has shown to be ancestrally determined by the male monopoly of tools and weapons, assuring the male group privileged access to resources, consequently exploiting women's labor, including procreation. This sexual-economic exchange is millennial, pre-dates capitalism, and while prostitution is an old part of it, surrogacy is a new one (though male appropriation of children is not new). To evaluate this stated parallel for outlining a public policy, there are theoretical and practical considerations to make. In general, public debates around issues of the "use" of women's sexual capacities polarize around two extreme theoretical visions. One is a paternalistic prohibition of "immoral" (though consensual) acts, motivated by the protection of the family created by marriage and by the defense of women's dignity. The other is an acceptance of the progressive commodification of these capacities stemming from capitalist/neoliberal ideology: its fetish of "individual choice" means renouncing to question and fight the context of inequality in which these choices are made.

What do women involved in these activities want for themselves? Not always do surrogates and prostitutes ask for a recognition of their activity as a job. Some prostitutes affirm that they are sex workers, while others consider the sex that brings them money only as a resource to be utilized promiscuously instead of participating in the marriage market or in the labor market. In the case of surrogates, they generally deny that surrogacy is just a job. But the problem is once again how women's work is socially considered:

> However, the other surrogates did not concur with SD2's opinion since they did not conceptualize surrogacy as a form of work. Their opinions reflected the conventional understanding of what is perceived as work. The work that is traditionally assigned to a woman, be it housework or reproductive labour, is invisibilized and devalued [in India and also elsewhere]. (Sama 2012, 55)

An unusual voice of a surrogate from India did claim an official recognition of her reproductive work for money:

> Women in our country will continue to do this, whether the government likes it or not. This is the best option available for many of us. If the government declares this to be a bad thing, we will do this in hiding, like prisoners, ashamed and weeping over our misfortune. If they declare this "a good thing," we will do it with the support of our family and neighbors, with our children next to us. We still won't sing about it proudly or yell it out to our neighbours, but we will do it with some normalcy...
> ...I might not be as educated as you are, but I do understand one thing: too many people gain from this surrogacy. [...] Our government must be getting something too. They would not want this to stop. All they will do is decide who gets more and who gets less in this business. (Pande 2014, 180–181).

But India, as we saw, is probably not bound to consider what these women are doing as work, and their stigma is not something peculiar to surrogacy but the same "whore stigma" attached to extramarital sex and therefore to pregnancy—though it could be in fact neutralized by the knowledge that no sexual relations are involved in surrogacy. Amrita Pande finds that the situation for workers in surrogacy is in fact getting better:

> Over the six years of my fieldwork, gradual shifts in the nature of resistances and negotiations become visible. As media coverage of the clinic and surrogacy increases, the stigma of surrogacy starts getting diluted, and women, especially the repeat surrogates, start negotiating higher payments and more support from their families and start demanding less interference by brokers. (Pande 2014, 11)

But there are some elements other than subjectivities that must be considered in expressing both a judgment in terms of public policy and also a moral judgment on these "bad women." The first element is akin to sex work and surrogacy: the suspension of *habeas corpus* on intimate life. Even though it is paradoxical, the use of one's sexual capacities for the exclusive sexual satisfaction of others in prostitution does not clash with the principle of sexual self-determination (at least not in formal terms). If we substantially look at sexuality *per se*, it is evident that the client is taking advantage of the prostitute's sexual capacities (this sad situation is not peculiar to sex work, being only but a part of the much broader sexual-economic exchange), and he is exploiting her, as employers do to their employees:

> It is not that the prostitution contract allows the client to buy the *person* of the prostitute while the employment contract merely allows the employer to buy the worker's fully alienable labor power. Both contracts transfer powers of command from seller to buyer (the extent of those powers and the terms of the transfer being the subject of the contract), and so require the seller to temporarily surrender or suspend aspects of her will. (O'Connell Davidson 2002).

Mutatis mutandis, the same considerations apply to surrogacy. The second element shows a different social consideration of these activities, a consideration which could conflate or diverge. The common view of prostitution condemns a woman not because she specifically "sells herself," but because she makes an unauthorized use of her sexual capacities (unauthorized by the dominant forces in society, and especially by religions), be it for money or for free. This view has been consolidating for millennia, and it is detrimental to all women, as it configures the notorious "Whore/Madonna" dichotomy, which undermines women's social and sexual free expression. (Only recently, the buyers of sexual services have also been subject to a similar stigma, e.g. in Swedish law.) Surrogacy is something new, and its public view is still uncertain. Public opinion does not condone the buyers of babies, but surrogacy cloaks itself under the rhetorical mantel of the happiness in giving and receiving a child—a very idealized notion of parenthood—and of the free choice of the birth mother to sign rational contracts.

The third element is decisive: the issue of privacy is the reason the Illuminist jurist Cesare Beccaria deemed prostitution "a victimless crime," decrying the prohibition inscribed in the laws of his time, as in the exchange of sex for money only the consent[141] of the people involved matters: they do no harm to anybody else—while to have a baby is the less private act that I can think of. Surrogacy considered as work amounts to baby-selling, while if sex work is voluntary, it should remain within the autonomy sphere. So the conclusions in terms of public policy must be different for the two.

Concerning prostitution, I believe that in the present circumstances the fight against sex workers' stigmatization is the most important route to take. Violence against sex workers is legitimized by social norms unjustly depriving them of human dignity because of what they do for a living, while this situation is unparalleled in surrogacy, where women have sometimes died because something went wrong during the pregnancy, but were never purposefully and hatefully assassinated. There is another important difference: paid surrogates are stigmatized in some parts of the world, but prostitutes are stigmatized everywhere. The ancient profound reason is that their sexual activity goes against the strict rules governing—or rather denying—women's sexuality, be it for money or for pleasure. A legalization of sex work would combat the whore stigma, broadening women's sexual freedom, as a normalization of the prostitute's activity (including respect and gratefulness by clients) would—somehow paradoxically—foster a freer view of women's sexuality. On the other hand, a regulation and normalization of surrogacy would just foster a market in babies. If surrogacy is considered as work, it is the job of producing a baby to be sold. One thing is what to do with one's own body, but another is what to do with a newborn. Plus, commodification in these two areas cannot be compared: the market for prostitution is huge, it would be impossible, as the abolitionists want, to prosecute all the existing clients—qualified as men from every walk of life. Neither is it possible to stop prostitution by outlawing it: in fact it is already outlawed in many states,

---

[141] The conditions of inequality in which consent is expressed always makes it seem somehow forced: only social and economic equality will free the subject from all forms of coercion. But even if consent is seldom free from economic and cultural coercion, if expressed by informed adults it must be taken for what it is (even with a false consciousness).

with no other result than worsening the social condition and consideration of sex workers. In history, even the harshest punishments assigned to prostitutes could not stop the illicit exchange. It is also a real question of privacy: the exchange takes place between consenting parties in private or secluded spaces. Forbidden sexual acts can easily be performed in the dark and in hiding, even with more gusto. Quite the contrary for surrogacy: it is still not so wide-spread, public opinion is instinctively against its baby-selling aspect, and it can effectively be prohibited without generating black markets: a pregnancy is difficult to hide and the product of this market is not a concealable object or an invisible service, but a human being whose birth must be registered and accounted for. Herbert Krimmel answers this way concerning the fear of a black market in surrogacy:

> Unlike users of alcohol, surrogacy is unlikely ever to have a large constituency. Therefore, rather than posing a difficult case, it seems like an ideal example of the type of behaviour that society should be able to effectively suppress. In fact, it is hard to imagine what could be a better example than surrogacy. (Krimmel 1992, 11)

Surrogacy needs public recognition and formal and informal approval: the wealthy parents who want to invest their money in having someone else manufacturing their children are not likely to let them live socially and legally unrecognized. Moreover, in prostitution there is no need for any particular technology, while gestational surrogacy, in its most controversial form, needs labs and the work of clinicians, subject to regulation. The culture of surrogacy is something new, it is fostered by the relative novelty of ART (that some countries have effectively banned inside their borders), and it has not yet spread all over the world, as the idea of prostitution since millennia has. But the role of third parties organizing prostitution and surrogacy is again similar.

Money making

Other actors are generally present on the scene of surrogacy: clinics, lawyers, agencies: they are clearly in it for the money coming from the intended parents. It is ironic that women's labor is mostly not paid but "reimbursed," while everybody else's is: doctors, lawyers, go-betweens—they all take a large share of the intended parents' savings. But if the birth mother cannot gain from her agreement, much less should other people be allowed to do so.

In California, according to a lawyer interviewed: "people who are making money are the agencies and the insurance companies," since they have created specific policies for surrogate mothers, at the enormous cost of $ 30,000:

> Usually, in the past, when I started this, you just bought a health care policy and it covered the surrogacy, the pregnancy and the birth, just like the regular persons. When surrogacy became more common, they had more and more buying an insurance policy for one year, paying the premium for a year. (Personal interview with lawyer, January 2013)

What do the agencies do? They are employment agencies and "womb hunters:"

> The agency fee is $10,000. This is due and payable in 4 installments.
> This fee is paid to utilize our services relating to your surrogate journey. This will cover advertising, interviewing, approving, and screening your surrogate mother. Completion of a background check for the surrogate and her husband, if applicable, as well as the in-home visit and interview is included in our fee. We will refer and coordinate the selection of fertility specialists, lawyers and psychologists as needed. We also will attend selected medical appointments upon request, support you and your surrogate mother, manage escrow disbursements, and manage your case from inception to birth and beyond.[142]

Agencies in the US are arranging contracts, finding egg donors and surrogates, and offering medical, legal, and psychological services to all parties involved. Doctors and lawyers also counsel prospective parents about the various possible reactions of all parties that can arise from the situation, and about the medical decisions to be taken, for example, agreements about "embryo reduction" should be made beforehand to avoid conflicts.

In the UK, where intermediation is forbidden, there are only non-profit "agencies," or rather associations, that are mainly based on volunteer work. COTS has about 750 members, and the fee to join is 850 GBP. It also declares that it receives many donations that permit this "reasonable membership fee." Surrogacy UK asks for the first 800 GBP and 50 GBP for each subsequent year. The money collected is spent on meetings, overhead costs, website and so on—I am sure that nobody gets rich.

But early testimonies on the role of intermediaries are upsetting:

---

[142] http://www.supportiveconceptionssurrogacy.com/financial-information.html accessed 1.1.2015.

> Debbie: The broker threatened me. He said they'll make things really hard for me to keep my baby. He didn't get explicit—but I knew he'd threatened other surrogate mothers. One surrogate said he had threatened to get her husband fired. Another surrogate said this guy could make your life absolute hell. He'd have a battery of lawyers against you. He'd make sure you had to pay every penny back or get you into jail if you couldn't pay it back fast enough. The broker told me that he had a hunch I was on welfare and that he was going to check the county welfare records and report me for trying to earn money as a surrogate if I backed out of the deal. (Chesler 1988, 62)

Elizabeth Kane described a very negative role of the agencies, too:

> There are 23 baby brokers in the United States and they are only interested in surrogate mothers as reproductive toys. The evidence is the number of women who are super ovulated 'to save the couple time and money' and the women who are accepted into their programs with multiple sclerosis, debilitating back problems and congenital heart defects. One surrogate mother from Texas with a heart condition was found dead in her bed on October 30, 1987. (Kane 1989)

To read agency announcements advertising their surrogates is disquieting:

> Currently represented by Your Family Creations this amazing woman comes with experience and passion as a gestational surrogate. Previously a GS [gestational surrogate] for triplets and one single baby both of which were incredibly positive & healthy pregnancies. Both experiences resulted in healthy deliveries.

Agencies are also working emotionally to reassure the surrogate mothers, as it is very evident in the autobiographical book by Kim Cotton on her experience. Cotton had a very good and sustaining relationship with the woman who followed her case on behalf of the US agency who managed this very first British surrogacy contract:

> A surrogate needs a positive relationship with the people she is helping. I believe it is important for the surrogate's emotional health. [...] There will always be a need for COTS, regardless of the problems over the years, because otherwise people will take a DIY approach without any advice or counselling. For every disaster there are many more success stories that people never hear about. (Wheathers 2008)

Janice Ciccarelli and Linda Beckman reviewed the 27 empirical studies on surrogacy published in 1983–2003, finding that sustained contact with the intended parents was important for a good outcome of the agreement, plus counseling:

> Ciccarelli's (1997) research was a follow-up study in which 14 participants (7 traditional surrogates and 7 gestational surrogates) were interviewed 5 to 10 years after serving as surrogate mothers. The surrogates were identified through surrogacy agencies with which the surrogates had worked, and were selected based on their willingness to voluntarily participate in the study. [...] Nevertheless, pre- and post-birth experiences, relationship with the contracting couple, and whether expectations about surrogacy are met,

> are important influences on the surrogate mothers' level of satisfaction [...] Unmet expectations are associated with dissatisfaction with the surrogacy experience. In Ciccarelli's (1997) study, 4 of 14 women had unmet expectations and, in two of these cases, expectations regarding level of closeness with the couple were not met. Such unmet expectations can arise at any time during the initial surrogacy arrangements, pregnancy, or many years post birth (Ciccarelli, 1997). Couple interaction with the surrogate immediately post birth appears important. If the surrogate mother is allowed to see and hold the baby and she feels she is being treated with respect, her satisfaction level is high (Hohman & Hagan, 2001) [...] Most surrogate mothers have some limited contact with the social parents (e.g., pictures of the child, telephone calls) for several years after the birth. Long-term satisfaction continues to depend on the surrogate mother's relationship with the couple and whether her expectations about the relationship and types of contact with the couple and child are met. (Ciccarelli and Beckham 2005, 31–32)

The problems found in studies were considered by the authors due to lack of "professional support:"

> Blyth (1994) identified 2 out of 17 women who regretted their decision. His is also the only study that reports a significant minority of women (about 25%) who experienced significant emotional distress in giving up the child. It is unclear whether the dissatisfaction stems from the surrogacy process itself, the lack of therapeutic intervention, or both. The considerable proportion of emotionally distressed and dissatisfied women may be exacerbated by the lack of professional support for women in Great Britain, where surrogacy agencies are illegal. (Ciccarelli and Beckham 2005, 33–34)[143]

Agencies structure the experience emphasizing the surrogate's responsibility to the couple, who—not really knowing her since they were introduced by the agencies—fears that she will not relinquish the child:

> Programs therefore openly address this issue with their surrogates, emphasizing that keeping the child would constitute an egregious act, reminding them that keeping the baby would constitute a terrible, perhaps even insurmountable blow to the lives of these emotionally exhausted and vulnerable couples. (Ragoné 1994, 40)

---

[143] Ciccarelli, J. C. (1997). *The surrogate mother: A post-birth follow-up study.* Unpublished Doctoral Dissertation. Los Angeles: California School of Professional Psychology.
Hohman, M. M., & Hagan, C. B. (2001). Satisfaction with surrogate mothering: A relational model. In *Journal of Human Behavior in the Social Environment*, 4, 61–84.
Blyth, E. (1994). "I wanted to be interesting. I wanted to be able to say 'I've done something with my life':" Interviews with surrogate mothers in Britain." In *Journal of Reproductive and Infant Psychology*, 12, 189–198.

An interviewed director of an agency says:

> "The surrogate bonds with the couple and not the baby; when the surrogate gives up the baby, she doesn't feel separation anxiety from giving up the baby but from losing her couple." None of this is left to chance, as discussed in Chapter 1. It is carefully planned by the programs. The semi-monthly or monthly therapy offered by the open programs (mandatory in some of them) is designed to maintain the desired state of mind or attitude toward the process. (Ragoné 1994, 79)

Ragoné also highlights that agencies in the US construct the surrogacy experience in a culturally palatable way:

> Casting surrogacy as the ultimate act of love serves to counteract conventional or traditionally held views that to keep and nurture the child is the best way to show love to a child to whom one has given birth. The following statement by a surrogate, with its almost fairy tale or mythic quality, is fairly common: "Twenty years from now I want to say, long ago I had a baby for someone who wanted a child very much. I hope he will grow up realizing how special he is. I hope he will know that there is a woman out there who cared enough to have him and give him up." (Ragoné 1994, 40)

The same dynamic is sustained by not-for-profit agencies:

> *Will my surrogate want to keep the child?*
> Surrogates never see the baby they are carrying for a couple as theirs—they have become involved in surrogacy because they want to help a couple have their own child. But it is important to realise that in the eyes of the law, the baby is not yours until the Parental Order has been issued after the baby is born: that means the surrogate could keep the baby if she chose to. That's why it is so important that surrogacy is based on friendship. No surrogate has ever tried to keep the baby for herself at Surrogacy UK and we firmly believe it is because we put such a strong emphasis on building a solid friendship first" (http://www.surrogacyuk.org/intended_parents/your-questions-answered accessed 12.10.2014).

Commercial agencies share the view that a surrogate mother is just a vessel for somebody else's child. In websites that advertise for surrogacy—not surprisingly—the "carrying" mother is completely erased from the description of the biological process of procreation:

> Same-sex couples face different fertility options and issues from heterosexual couples who can attempt conception without any medical help. Lesbian couples require an outside source of sperm while gay men require both eggs and uterus.[144]

Of course this parallels the situation of the bought "workforce" that cannot be detached from the person of the worker, as uteruses generally need attachment to a woman to be able to work. The imaginary reduction of a

---

[144] *Same-sex Couples & Fertility*: http://abivf.com/patients/same-sex, accessed 15.6.2013

woman to her reproductive parts becomes logical if we consider that the message from the agencies is aimed at intended parents, who are their source of profit while the surrogate mothers are just the means to get it.

The role of emotional support after all is not that different with or without a binding contract, Elizabeth Anderson even finds it more deceptive if the contract is not valid:

> Since it [the agency] could not rely on the law to enforce the adoptive parents' wishes regardless of the surrogate's feelings, it would have to make sure that she assumed the perspective which it and its clients have of her: as "rented plumbing." (Anderson 1990, 88)

It seems that without formal or informal "counseling" it is very difficult for surrogacy to work:

> Programs (usually closed) that dispense with the need for the various kinds of psychological reinforcement provided by the open programs are thus more likely to encounter surrogates who desire to keep the child. (Ragoné 1994, 78)

Even though it does not mean that all women who suffer are keeping their children. Stella and Pam for example worked for a program that went bankrupt: they were told that it was their own option to go on with surrogacy or to "discontinuing the contract." "Some option," they commented, "what choice did we have? We were pregnant." All surrogates were left without counseling:

> Stella said: "I first saw the baby again at two weeks and it was really hard, I cried and cried. The pain was really intense, but I never regretted doing this." Pam, another Smith program ex-surrogate, stated: "You have nine months with the child, but it's how you choose to handle those feelings that counts. There will be a tremendous amount of grief and sadness and yet it's not right for me to raise this child. I don't have the energy. If it wasn't for this couple wanting this child, I wouldn't be pregnant. There are nights I wake up crying and I see this is going to be hard" (Ragoné 1994, 78 and 79)

What to think of the psychologists and counselors couching the surrogates about the baby not being theirs? Do they find it ethical to reinforce such an attitude? Do the professional orders find it unquestionable? The practice sounds like brainwashing, and if it is judged necessary for a good outcome of the surrogacy agreement, this implies that the will of the mother is not considered to suffice.

Another typical example of the disavowal of the point of view of surrogate mothers is the representation by third parties of her possible decision to keep the baby as a "risk," or even "unsafe:"

> Since common law presumes that the woman giving birth is the child(ren)'s mother, surrogacy requires extensive legal assistance so that the Intended Parents are recognized as such on the birth certificate and a drawn-out custody battle is avoided. Whereas the legal status of gestational surrogacy is well established in California and several other states, traditional surrogacy presents more legal pitfalls because the surrogate's claim to the child(ren) is much stronger since it is based upon both a genetic and gestational link. Thus, for safety reasons alone, gestational surrogacy is generally preferable to traditional surrogacy (Alta Bates IVF Program, http://abivf.com/solutions/surrogacy, accessed 17.2.2015).

The "risks of surrogacy" even to intended parents are that the mother might feel attachment to her baby and want to keep it, a fact that the intended parents should instead regard as legitimate, one of the numerous risks of not obtaining a healthy child at the end of the gestational process. Instead the only risk they contemplate is that the surrogate "reneges on the agreement." The birth mother is not a human being but a human factory. The fact that a possible conflict about parental rights is framed by the contract, by the rhetoric of the agencies, and in much of the literature[145] in terms of "risk" for the intended parents, completely disregards the primary position of the birth mother in relation to the newborn. This reflects an ideology of the superiority of genetics to flesh and blood ties, perhaps reflecting the fact that fatherhood is always based just on those, or maybe just as a consequence of the validity of the contract. The German documentary *Dein Bauch—mein Baby!* (Your belly my baby, 2011) by Focus TV features a woman doctor in Ukraine who openly declares: "The surrogate mother should not be able to develop maternal feelings for the baby." The intended mother explains: "Following the doctor's advice, we did not let her be nursed. For the girl, it would have been better, but worse for the construction of an emotive bond between me and her."

This documentary shows the intended parents watching the surrogate mother in birthing pain, then receiving the child to go home with. In the end, the Ukrainian woman declares to have done all this only for her kids, cashing in 15,000 euros. The intended father concludes: "I would do it again.

---

[145] E.g, in an essay on the Chimera of "homoparentality" we find these risks: "More than 85% of the families of gay fathers were formed through adoption. Obviously, it is more difficult for a gay male to have a biological child than for a lesbian to have one, finding a woman who is willing to be a surrogate mother is much more difficult than finding a sperm donor. The risks of surrogacy are great; some states do not recognize contracts between prospective parents and surrogates, and the media abound in stories like the Mary Beth Whitehead case, where a surrogate mother reneged on her agreement and sought custody of the child" (Johnson and O'Connor 2002, 97).

It is no question of right or wrong," suggesting that having his own baby was of such paramount importance so as to numb or skip altogether any moral judgment. There can be consequences of this attitude:

> In 2009, [in India] a young surrogate started suffering from uncontrollable bleeding just a few days after delivering the baby. The clinic—unprepared for complications, told her husband to book his own ambulance to a nearby hospital. The woman died on the way to the hospital. Not surprisingly, neither the clinic nor the intended parents were ready to take responsibility for the young woman's death. In a similar case in 2012, a surrogate collapsed due to "unexplained complications" in the eighth month of her pregnancy. The clinic was able to perform an emergency surgery and save the baby. (Pande 2014, 14–15)

How many thousand dollars is a woman's life worth? With or without caps, the "reimbursement" for these "amazing women" changed very little in the US in the first two decades:

> surrogates receive between 10,000 and 15,000 USD (for three to four months of insemination and nine months of pregnancy, on average), a fee that has changed only nominally since the early 80s. As one program psychologist explained, the amount paid to surrogates is intentionally held at an artificially low rate by the programs so as to screen out women who might be motivated solely by monetary gain. (Ragoné 1996, 354)

Since then, market forces must have been at work as the price has gone up to 20–25,000 USD. Many announcements of prospective surrogates stress their experience and professionalization, asking for a correspondingly higher remuneration, e.g.: "Since I am already a proven surrogate my compensation base fee is $35k plus normal expenses (legal, maternity clothes, etc.)." Agencies are promising even more: "Illinois is one of the best states in America to be a surrogate mother & our surrogates earn up to $45k PLUS expenses! Find out why & apply today for FREE!"[146] Agencies are sometimes welcomed by surrogates because dealing seems to be a difficult terrain for them:

> The most difficult topic of any surrogacy agreement is—anything to do with money! A LOT of surrogates are not comfortable discussing this with potential IP's and prefer to turn to an agency for help. A first-time surrogate's compensation ranges from compassionate (unpaid) arrangements, which are few, to $25,000.00. What are you comfortable with as far as compensation is concerned? Remember that your family is MOST important when making that decision. I have talked to surrogates who state "It's not about the money." Which is ultimately great, it should not be about the money. What it should be about is your family. (Alexander 2006, 39)

---

[146] http://www.illinoissurrogateagency.com accessed 13.07.2013.

So, how much does a surrogacy agreement cost to intended parents? In California, where there is no price cap, costs are calculated between 80,000 and 120,000 USD,[147] but Ragoné (1994, 34) relates of gestational surrogacies costing 200,000 and more. In Israel: "In practice, payments to the surrogate are currently around 35–45,000 USD, with a total cost of 50–75,000 in unmediated agreements, and approximately an extra 10,000 in mediated ones" (Shakargy 2013, 238). The Israeli Guidelines describe the compensation as including, but not limited to: pain and suffering, discomfort, loss of income, travel, clothing, household help and childcare, plus ten hours of separate legal counseling. In Thailand the total price is 36,000 USD. In Ukraine the cost is between 30,000 and 45,000 USD, in Greece 14,000–50,000 EUR, in India 22,000–35,000 USD. There are even cheaper places. In South Africa a surrogacy (only for residents) costs 200,000 rand (about 17,400 USD). In Russia the "services" of a surrogate mother cost (at least) about 20,000 USD, more if there are intermediaries. Just 25,000 USD are asked by an Indian clinic for a complete package with all guarantees for success: sperm would be collected from the intended father (popularly called "sperm on a rickshaw") and the clinic will keep on trying with different eggs and different surrogates until a pregnancy is established (Hochschild 2012, 86). This might involve using more than one surrogate at a time, "and if both become pregnant, it can happen that the client insists that one must abort" (Andersen 2013). A sum close to the Indian package deal was requested by a Russian agency with an office in Kiev: the charge would have been 24,000 EUR for just one attempt, and 30,000 for unlimited attempts (documentary *Dein Bauch—mein Baby!* 2011).

In India the clinics determine the price and women or their families rarely bargain about it. The individualized price is a source of animosity: "One dismayed surrogate carrying twins for an Indian couple discovered that she was being paid far less—$3,400—than the surrogate sleeping in the next cot, who was carrying a single baby for an American couple for $5,000"

---

[147] A Facebook post sums the current costs up: "I don't think I've ever heard of a US surrogacy journey costing $50k, the cheapest is around $75k and we spent a LOT more than that!! so to break down the costs a bit—IVF (full package with multiple cycles) ranges from $35-50k, surrogate fee ranges from $20-30k, egg donor ranges from $5-10k, legal fees range from $5-10k the killer then comes in using an agency which can be from $15-50k and then health insurance which can be from $10-100k...!!!! so it all adds up - that doesn't include travel or incidentals or anything on top!!!"

(Hochschild 2012, 91). Failed attempts are rewarded with nothing. Other sources place the remuneration for surrogates between 2 and 8,000 USD, while the yearly mean income in India is 1,500 USD. But this great sum is not at all sufficient to really change the lives of the surrogates, especially given that health care is private, so sooner or later all savings end up there (Pande 2014, 190 ff.).

In the UK the sum to pay to the surrogate varies between 12,000 and 15,000 GBP, and a non-profit agency openly considers it as compensation for work:

> Let's be straight: UK surrogates do get paid. Some surrogates have their actual out of pocket expenses covered, which can be no small amount once you add up travel costs, loss of earnings, extra childcare, medications, support with housekeeping and additional food costs. More commonly, UK surrogates agree to be paid a lump sum, including expenses but in a fairly general way without much reference to the actual costs. Figures of £12,000 to £15,000 are typical (often with variable costs like travel and loss of earnings in addition) plus other payments if the surrogate miscarries or delivers twins. We are also aware that some UK surrogates (particularly those advertising their services online) are charging £20,000 or even more. None of this is new, with such arrangements being common in the UK for at least 20 years.[148]

All the listed remunerations are rewarding from an economic point of view for the prospective mothers. In fact, both in low income countries, as India, in middle-income ones, such as Ukraine, the fee paid to the surrogate mother amounts to much more than the yearly revenue for a low income job, which in the rich countries is instead the standard fee for a newbie (20–25,000 USD in the US, 10–15,000 GBP in the UK), a sum that is not considered despicable:

> The going rate for surrogacy in the US is 25,000 to 35,000 for first time surrogates. I can't think of a single job I can get right now that pays that with my education and experience. Plus I can work while being a surrogate! Now that is just here in the US, but as a "poor" person I think that is pretty great. (Comment posted in http://rhrealitycheck.org/article/2014/04/23/invoking-choice-discussing-surrogacy-feminist-concern-mistake/ accessed 28.12.2014).

Though the reimbursement is paid in installments, the biggest chunk is generally pocketed at delivery: so much the fiction of paying the "gestational services" and not for the child itself.

---

[148] http://www.brilliantbeginnings.co.uk/blog/how-much-can-uk-surrogates-get-paid dated 30 September 2014, accessed 1.12.2014.

Limiting the remuneration to the reimbursement of expenses in order to avoid creating a market for babies has not succeeded, also because many women in fact like the job, that they find more suitable than other low-skilled occupations as it allows them to be a stay-at-home mom. It is certainly true that human feelings and the exchange of money on a market can go hand in hand (provided the "private money" is culturally distinguished)—but who is emotionally gaining from this and who is emotionally exploited? Many birth mothers crumbled at the discover that the intended parents they so generously helped were just exploiting them, waiting for the delivery of the baby to disappear from their lives. And this is just one of the possible conflictual points in their relationship.

Relationships and conflicts

Money aside, other social exchanges are taking place in surrogacy, like status acquisition by the birth mother having helped the infertile, both in her own eyes and in pro-natalist societies at large. But the recognition for what she does as an act of generosity is far from universal. It might be affine to the Christian spirit, but in India to the contrary she must hide, risking her reputation. An incentive for Indian surrogates are the further obligations that they hope the intended parents will recognize for their deed. Kalindi Vora (2013, see also Pande 2014) in her ethnographic research at the Manushi clinic writes extensively about the hope of the surrogate mothers to benefit from the bond with the rich couple, being further economically helped by them, even brought to live in a richer country. They consider that what they gave them, a human life, cannot simply be equated with a sum of money. But establishing a permanent bond with further obligations is discouraged by the clinic, and it is likely to remain a fantasy. For Pande this is again a set-up to exploit the women:

> The (often fictive) relationships formed with intended parents downplay the contractual and business aspect of surrogacy and further undermine the surrogates' ability to view themselves as workers and to defend their interests as such. [...] The good surrogate hesitates to negotiate the payment and instead treats it as God's gift to her to fulfill her familial responsibilities. (Pande 2014, 14 and 23)

What is the experience of the intended parents? I could not directly interview any in the US—though I did have discussions with some in Italy.

> It definitely grows each year. When I first started doing this, there were probably three or four attorneys, and now it's improved, there are probably about 30. It is very good with the IVF, that's why it's becoming so successful and lots of people are doing this and that's why more people, women, are putting off pregnancy until they're too old, because of working. By the time they want a baby they are in their 40s. (Personal interview, January 2013)

Earlier in the interview she had described the intended parents more sympathetically:

> Usually, people start by being infertile. Usually, parents using surrogates are people who have had years of miscarriage and infertility and nothing has worked, it's not just somebody who said I don't wanna be pregnant, I wanna be a parent, nothing like that. It's infertile people desperate to have a baby. (Personal interview, January 2013)

The Berkeley gynecologist declares that the clinic he works for only accepts infertile women:

> I think that we don't like the idea that someone is going to use a surrogate just in order to avoid getting pregnant and fat.
> *Q: Because you think she will not be able to mother?*
> A: I think that most women who want to have children, may also want the experience of pregnancy, that's kind of logical. (Personal interview, January 2013)

Elizabeth Kane had no pity:

> Many couples are in their second and third marriage, are middle aged and wealthy. Paying a baby broker $12,000 to $15,000 to find them a healthy uterus is not a financial strain. Many times the wife is surgically infertile by choice and already has children from a previous marriage. Her husband is not childless but is a step father to her children. Only because he is obsessed with exercising his "right to procreate," must his wife submit to his desires to hire a surrogate wife if she wants to preserve their marriage. She too is being intimidated and coerced into signing a contract to have her husband's procreative demands met by another woman. (Kane 1989)

Janice Raymond recounts the answer in court of an intended mother when asked about how she had experienced the arrangement: "Since she had testified several minutes before about the great merits of surrogacy, many were shocked as she sobbed: 'It's so humiliating to have my husband ask a strange woman to bear his child'" (Raymond 1994, xxviii).

Where surrogacy contracts are enforceable, they are formulated in ways that make intended parents feel it in their own right to make decisions about the pregnant woman's health, even about abortion or embryo reduction. Not only do they pay the surrogate mother, but they also buy her a health insurance—usually in the United States these women are among the dozen of millions that do not possess one, while in India only rich women use medical assistance for birthing and can afford to do so. So the intended parents expect the surrogate to comply with the contract by obeying the medical directions on how to conduct her pregnancy and the related aspects of her life (that is: her life) in the supposed best way for the developing child, such as not having sexual relationships until pregnant and often also afterwards, or eating only a particular kind of healthy food on one hand, while submitting to all kinds of drugs and examinations on the other—e.g. amniocentesis for young women is not only dangerous but totally useless. The Berkeley gynecologist put it bluntly: "It's not their pregnancy, not a thing they can make a decision about"—a view not so different from the Indian one. The current template for a Californian surrogacy contract specifies the details of what the gynecologist meant:

> The Surrogate agrees not to smoke any type of cigarettes, drink alcoholic beverages or excessive caffeinated beverages, or to use any illegal drugs, prescription or non-prescription drugs without the written consent of her physician and/or obstetrician.
> The Surrogate agrees not to travel outside of the United States of America after the second trimester of the pregnancy, with the exception of the event of an extreme illness or death in the Surrogate's family and only upon the written consent of her physician and/or obstetrician. [...]
> The Surrogate and Surrogate's Husband agree to make no attempt to contact or maintain communications with the Child(ren) born pursuant to this Agreement, or with any member of the stated Parties' families subsequent to the birth of the Child(ren) without the Genetic Father or Intended Mother's prior written approval. Further, Surrogate and Surrogate's Husband agree that they will not intervene or interfere with the upbringing of the Child(ren), or in the lives of the Genetic Father, Intended Mother and Child(ren), unless otherwise agreed in writing and signed by all Parties.
> In the event that custody of the Child(ren) is awarded to the Surrogate or her family, or any individual or organization not related to the Genetic Father, by any court decision or otherwise, the Genetic Father shall be indemnified by the Surrogate for any and all moneys he is required to pay for child support or medical procedure related expenses pursuant to any court order, and shall be entitled to immediate reimbursement from the Surrogate for all allowable reasonable and actual expenses paid by the Genetic Father and Intended Mother to the Surrogate pursuant to this Agreement or expended on behalf of the Surrogate.[149]

Clauses on abortion and selective termination follow, with the same peremptory tone. Conversely, the template clauses for a traditional surrogacy contract should be more convincing than threatening, and in fact they appeal to good feelings:

---

[149] *Sample GS Contract*: www.allaboutsurrogacy.com/sample_contracts/GScontract1.htm accessed 22.1.2015.

> The Surrogate and her Husband understand that the Intended Parents have waited many years and are now expending significant time and financial resources to bring a child into their home, and are now relying greatly on the Surrogate to carry their Child. It is also understood by the Parties that grave, severe and intense emotional distress, humiliation and mental anguish may occur to either of the Parties as a result of an uncured or incurable material breach by the other Party, and the breaching Party may be held liable for such emotional distress, humiliation and mental anguish as well as other legal and equitable remedies, under one or more legal theories.[150]

To guarantee the goal, not only emotional pressure, but also lying to surrogate mothers appears sometimes necessary: in India women were not told that their commissioning couples are gay, in the US a previous voluntary abortion of an intended mother was canceled from the file shown to the surrogate, and the fact that the intended mother was not infertile was discovered too late by another surrogate, as Smerdon, Ragoné and Pande recount. Ragoné concludes:

> Programs advise the couple about the importance of creating and maintaining the image of being a loving and devoted couple, who has the ideal marriage (except for their inability to have a child) and is ready to take a child into a perfect, idyllic home. (Ragoné 1994, 42)

Hilary Hanafin also found that the tie between adults is the most important thing: "It works for us because [the surrogate] cannot imagine hurting this couple whom she knows and likes so much" (quoted in Chesler 1988, 57). But the other way 'round is apparently not as common:

> Debbie: I thought my couple and I would always be the best of friends. I imagined we'd always spend our holidays together—just one big happy family. I can't believe that all along they planned to get rid of me once they had the baby.
> Helen: Even now it's really hard for me to admit that the whole thing was a setup against me from the start. I can't even complain about being paid too little for all my suffering. I was ready to do it for nothing. (Chesler 1988, 48)

Chesler adds: "most contract couples are very grateful to their surrogate mother. They also want nothing more to do with her after the baby is safely 'theirs'" (Chesler 1988, 60). A Spanish gay father states:

> I prefer the procedure of India, I mean the procedure where I think the role of the mother ismore in her place because, at least in couples I know who have done it in the United States, the mother [gestante] becomes like a person of the family, like an aunt, and I think roles get a little confused. (Smietana 2013, 212)

---

[150] *Sample TS Contract*: www.allaboutsurrogacy.com/sample_contracts/TScontract1.htm accessed 12.7. 2013

Accounts abound of the distance between birth mothers' and intended parents' assessment of the situation. Surrogates intend their engagement as a cooperative effort to dote an infertile couple with a baby:

> I was friends with this family and I wanted to help them, because I knew that I had easy pregnancies and I saw that they wanted it so much. [...] Money was not important, I would have done it for free, but they felt better knowing what I was putting my body and my family through to compensate me. You know it was more important for them to pay me than for me to receive it. (Bertschi 2014, 139)

But the intended parents (especially intended mothers, challenged in their role) usually have an utilitarian view, and they even think that paying to get a child from a poor country is fair trade: "Hiring a surrogate from a distant Third World nation was visualized as another form of development aid, with the hiring couple playing the role of brave missionaries battling all odds to help the needy" (Pande 2014, 101). The surrogates in Pande's work generally found that they were not treated with respect: after delivery, the couples they helped in establishing a family often just disappeared. Nevertheless, intended parents feel that they made a generous deal, and take pride in their "help," as this US intended father:

> We are happy to have been able to help the surrogate, because she was divorced. In India it is very difficult for a woman, and so she wanted to use the money to put her children through education and to start a business. So we are happy we have been able to help her and she has given us a wonderful family. (Bertschi 2014, 197)

Another intended father from the US so explains his choice of surrogacy over adoption: "Surrogacy offers you more control and you know that you are going to have a baby in the end, whereas with adoption, there aren't as many opportunities to control the outcome" (Bertschi 2014, 142). Why is it perceived to be easy? Probably because women do not count, and poor women are just walking incubators.

The rejection of disabled children is another issue shedding light on the intents of many "intended parents:" the eugenic dream of the perfect offspring. As the child comes delivered as a product, if it is defective some intended parents feel that the right thing to do is send it back to the producer (thought there is no guarantee of motherly love in a noncommercial birth either). Many cases have been reported by the press, a particularly sad one involving Baby Gammy, "commissioned" in Thailand by an Australian man pluriconvicted of child abuse together with his mail-order bride, whose embryos were implanted in a Thai woman. She gave birth to twins, one healthy and one disabled, but the couple only kept the healthy child abandoning the other. Outrage arose across the world, and the case prompted Thailand to outlaw surrogacy—though commercial surrogacy had already been forbidden by Thailand's Medical Council in 1997.

Gillian Goslinga-Roy finely analyzes the contrasting reasons to enter the agreement. Pamela is the intended mother, Julie the "carrier:"

> To Pamela's repeated "You baked her" and "Look at what a good job you did: she's beautiful," Julie insisted, over and over, through her tears, "look at the good job we did." Her own aspirations of this moment—the sense of having shared a pregnancy, of being a part of the making of a family, her desire for a deep and satisfying reciprocity—were lost in Pamela's completely utilitarian assessment of Julie having done the job well. (Goslinga-Roy 2000, 134)

Goslinga-Roy concludes:

> Pamela's anxieties and guilt, I have suggested, were greatly exacerbated by her uncritical dependence on a biologized notion of motherhood. This dependence, reinforced by the discourses and practices around her, precluded the possibility of a genuine sharing of the pregnancy, the comothering of sorts Julie was in fact proposing. Pamela's inability to expand the boundaries of her own privatized, individualized, and gendered self/body pitted her against the person of Julie, sometimes explicitly, sometimes implicitly (Goslinga-Roy 2000, 129).

Exploitation by the intended parents, according to Goslinga-Roy, did not happen because of the objective exchanges but because of culture—but this culture is the one legitimizing commodification of human relationships, and it is fostered by the current mode of production:

> All said and done, Julie ended up being a breeder for the Martins. But she did not become a breeder because she carried and gave birth to a baby that was not "her" own. Nor did she become a breeder because she was paid to carry this baby. Julie became a breeder because the Martins' own personal biographies, along with the discourse and practices of the assisted reproductive technologies, are seeped in a potent and heady cocktail of biogenetic and class ideologies and practices, a 350-year-old Euro-American brew called biopower by Foucault and biological embodiment by myself here, which made it virtually impossible for the Martins to even begin to comprehend Julie's expectations and desires or to see her as anything but a womb.
> The recipes for this brew are any number of rigidly unitary discourses and practices, such as the natural supremacy of the privatized nuclear family; the polite use of money to discharge moral obligations; the biologized notion of motherhood which suggests that women make babies inside their bodies, alone, and not within domestic networks; the naturalization, in our discourse, of a splintered reproduction into "genetic," "biological," and "social" aspects as though these exist in real life as distinct ontological domains; the pathologization of infertility as a condition of the body; the unselfconscious privileging of desire that is class... the list goes on and on. The essential ingredient, however, is the compelling ability of a privatized and fetishized discourse to dishonor real-time biography, ambiguity, multiplicity, and change.

> Julie was able to de-biologize motherhood for herself as well as deprivatize her body and thus aspire to a collective making of a child with another couple. If she failed in her vision, it was only because the Martins, supported by almost everything around them, refused to consider her and the work she did as a part of their collective body. (Goslinga-Roy 2000, 136–7)

The fantasies of the intended mother, in their utter absurdity, epitomize Goslinda-Roy's conclusions very well:

> Inside Julie's body, Pamela told me once, her child was alone and among strangers, "away from her parents who want to love her and hold her." She longed for the day her baby would come "home." (Goslinga-Roy 2000, 132)

The surrogate mother's feelings are often not reciprocated, as her presence can be a source of embarrassment once the family is constituted: "After a time they might cut you off" because "things change after birth," observes a US surrogate who had this experience (Bertschi 2014, 150). Kaytlin Alexander warns colleagues that future contact must be carefully negotiated:

> What are your expectations regarding contact before, during and after the birth? Would it be a deal-breaker for you if a couple stated that they only wanted communication via e-mail after the birth of the baby(ies)? If so, then you need to stand firm on your expectations.

But she gives no illusion that a good relationship will hold:

> But be aware of this—just because you expect it does not always mean that it will happen. You have to trust your own instinct when it comes to people to determine whether you feel the couple will stand by their word in the end [...] Prepare your heart for the possibility of broken promises. You may have heard or read about the many instances of couples promising their surrogates terms that sound like rainbows and sunshine. Unfortunately, in the end, all that some surrogates get is the rain. (Alexander 2006, 13)

The intended parents' couple interviewed by Hochschild were even surprised by her question about whether they would continue to see the surrogate:

> They imagined themselves as outsourcers paying a stranger to provide a professionally supervised service. They hoped to establish a pleasant, temporary bond with the surrogate, to pay her, thank her, and leave. They sought to create the sort of relationship one might establish with an obstetrician or dentist. (Hochschild 2012, 83)

They were also ignorant of the relationship between a birth mother and her newborn, as the intended mother later admitted: "When we were doing the surrogacy, I wasn't so aware of the mother-child bond. I didn't know a baby could recognize the voice of the mother who carried it. I guess I felt detached" (Hochschild 2012, 83). There is no shared culture about motherhood, only ignorance and taboos.

The literature records not only episodes of conflict around the delivery of the child, but also around other relations between the parties to the agreement. A surrogate mother complains on a forum about pressure in the choice of delivery:

> I want to go about labor and delivery as natural as possible and from the beginning they've sworn they trusted me and would back me up when it came to fighting for a vaginal, natural birth. Now IM [intended mother] is basically telling me that I'm lucky she's not scheduling an automatic c-section because the babies are hers, so she can decide how and when they're born.[151]

In 2006 litigation was started because of the intended parents' "businesslike" attitude—for example in planning not to say to their Asian kids that they had been borne by a white mother. The question of embryo reduction was decisive: "She was also reportedly angered when, after expressing her reservation about carrying a twin pregnancy, she was immediately scheduled for termination without further input or discussion" (Crokin 2010, case 639). This is another case of litigation, over abortion:

> When Helen Beasley, a 26-year-old single mother from Britain, agreed to serve as a surrogate for Charles Wheeler and Martha Berman [in 2002], she considered it an opportunity to provide the American couple with a "happy ending." Beasley did not anticipate that several months into the pregnancy she would find herself engaged in a legal battle over the terms of the surrogacy contract. What prompted the lawsuit was Beasley's discovery that she was carrying twins. This discovery led Wheeler and Berman, both lawyers in California, to terminate the contract, having paid Beasley only $ 1,000 of the $ 20,000 they had originally promised her. The couple relied on the terms of the surrogacy contract, which called for Beasley to abort additional fetuses in the event of a multiple pregnancy. When she refused to proceed with the selective reduction, Beasley filed a lawsuit against the couple, claiming that they had abandoned the children. In response, Wheeler and Berman demanded $80,000 in expenses, alleging that Beasley broke the terms of the surrogacy contract. [...] In the end, the court ordered the couple to pay Beasley $6,500 and to continue making payments to her in the future. (London 2012, 391 and n. 7)

Especially where the contract is legally valid, the few conflicts between surrogate mothers and intended parents reported by the press are usually conflicts around abortion.[152] Some women refuse to carry twins while others do

---

[151] http://www.allaboutsurrogacy.com/forums/index.php?showtopic=54547 accessed 6.2013.
[152] E.g. Bryan Robinson: "Fetuses and surrogacy lose in legal battle" (http://abcnews.go.com/US/sory?id=92627&page=1#.UeaKiaxpDZI accessed 15.7.2013); Mark Hughes: "'It

not want to intentionally abort, and the intended parents generally want to take this decision themselves. Nevertheless the pregnant woman is everywhere and always, without exception, the only one legally entitled to terminate a pregnancy. Some commentators are in favor of attributing the choice to abort embryos to the intended parents, with arguments configuring the future child as a property:

> Most legal and medical professionals believe, under the current state of the law, that a gestational carrier can freely abort the entrusted embryo at any time, and for any reason, without recourse for the intended parents. This is wrong. The gestational carrier should be treated as a fiduciary, the trustee of the embryo she is carrying. Her responsibilities as a fiduciary are to protect the subject of the trust, to defend the trust corpus from attack, to make the subject of the trust productive, to satisfy her duty of loyalty to all beneficiaries and to not engage in self-dealing. Any one of these duties alone would preclude the gestational carrier from getting an abortion unless her own life or physical health were at stake. (Yamamoto e Moore 2001, 185)

Or simply because the signed contract so commands:

> Although this provision may violate a woman's right to privacy, the surrogate mother is contracting to bear a child. Therefore, any abortion procedure for reasons other than to save the life of the mother will constitute a breach of the contract. (Garrity 2000, 829, n 105)

But the point at issue is not the woman's right to abort, constitutionally guaranteed, but the legality of the fines imposed by the contract if the woman exercises it without the approval of the intended parents or their doctor's. I am not aware of verdicts striking down these unconscionable clauses. Running away can be the only solution: much commented in the press was the flight of a pregnant woman to a US state that does not recognize surrogacy contracts:

> In one such case in Connecticut where a fetus was shown to have abnormalities, the surrogate was offered $10,000 to abort. She declined. Because state law clearly identified the "purchasers" as the parents, the surrogate moved to another state, had the baby and placed her in an adoptive home. (www.cnn.com/2013/03/04/health/surrogacy-kelley-legal-battle accessed 5.7.2013).

---

wasn't their decision to play God': Surrogate mother flees after couple demands abortion of disabled baby," The Daily Telegraph, National Post Wire Services 13.3.06 (http://news.nationalpost.com/2013/03/06/it-wasnt-their-decision-to-play-god-surrogate-mother-flees-after-couple-demands-abortion-of-disabled-baby/ accessed 15.7.2013); "Surrogate mother pushes for adoption," BBC, 12.8.2001, http://news.bbc.co.uk/2/hi/health/1485494.stm accessed 20.7.2013).

The mother herself described the sequence of events in her blog http://surrogateinsanity.blogspot.it/ (accessed 20.7.2013).

Also in California, where a contract is sacred, conflicts emerge about issues of control and abortion:

> *Q: Did you ever have a case where the surrogate tries to go against the Supreme Court?*
> A: Never. The only trouble I've run into is when the parents seem to be too controlling. It's the only time I've had issues. The surrogate says: "I don't want them at the medical appointments, I don't want them at the birth, I just can't take it anymore." And I had one time when somebody didn't want to be reduced, from triplets to twins, she really really didn't want to do it, but in the end she did it, because she knew she had agreed to at the time. You know, there's always a phrase there: "If there's a severe genetic defect, the parents have the right..." If you get a surrogate who is saying: "Well, I don't want to do it if...," then I tell the parents "I don't think it is a good match for you." If you find a surrogate and parents who would never abort, fine, that's a match. You have to really find people who psychologically match that way. (Personal interview, January 2013)

For the lawyer, the contract is not even decisive as there is a right of the father to his offspring, expressed in genetic terms:

> *Q: Shouldn't the surrogate not be bound by a contract? She should have a chance to change her mind.*
> A: No matter what, he's gonna be the father, because he's genetically related, 99% of the time. I see your point about coercion but that's why you make sure they are represented by a lawyer. Before they sign the contract, you make sure they have a lawyer who explains... The thing about having the contract, is that it makes you discuss and think about the outcomes: "What about if the parents want an abortion?" It makes you talk about abortion, it makes you talk about reduction, it makes you talk about things. The thing is: even if you didn't have a contract, it's legal and the law recognizes the [intended] parents.
> But the point is, it's not really the contract. I don't think it is making [stopping?] these people who really want to try to keep the baby. The few times they're trying to keep the baby in the court are when the parents are going to get divorced and they don't want the baby to get into a broken family.
> I talk to the surrogates, there's never a question in their minds about it, I've done it hundreds of times. I always say: "Look, are you sure? You're going to give this child," and they say: "Oh God no, I've got three kids, I don't want another kid. I just want to help these people." And the surrogates I've talked to they do it ... clearly... for them 20 or 30,000 dollars it's a lot of money, but that's not enough to carry a kid. They like to be pregnant, they like the feeling, they like the attention, the feeling of being pregnant. (Personal interview, January 2013)

The potential conflict on the issue of abortion is considered by the gynecologist as the most worrying factor of the entire procedure:

> And they [the intended parents who want to skip agencies] do not know about the criteria, how you go about evaluating if someone is going to be a good candidate for surrogacy. So, you know, the psychological, sociological perspective, medical perspective, you want to review their references, you do not rush into it.

> You don't want to form a bond between the intended parents and the surrogate before you know if the surrogate is going to be ok. I mean, the surrogate has to accept the idea that the parents may want to terminate the pregnancy and there are lots of people that are opposed to abortion, so you have to talk to them about it; or if there's an abnormality and maybe it's twins and the parents want to eliminate one of the children and keep the other one, you need to make sure that the person is going to be ok doing something that maybe they wouldn't do themselves in their own pregnancy. It's not their pregnancy, not a thing they can make a decision about, and that eliminates lots of people.
>
> *Q: What could be a cause for termination of pregnancy? Relationship problems?*
> A: Well, I mean, I think.. It depends, if the egg came from the woman… she's trying to get pregnant, she may be older and the egg may not be so healthy, so there are going to be significant chances that the surrogate is going to lose the pregnancy to a miscarriage; or if the pregnancy goes on and you do genetic testing, you may know the pregnancy is not normal and in that situation it may also not work out. In case in which you use the egg donor, then it's more likely to be successful, because usually the egg donors are young and the embryos are healthier and there's much less risk of miscarriage. But then it would be… for instance, when we work with gay men we use an egg donor and a surrogate, so we have an ideal egg and an ideal uterus, so the pregnancy is very likely to succeed. For each couple that came, that has been successful, and that's an ideal kind of situation, but if you're dealing with the egg from a woman who's maybe 39–40 years old, then maybe the pregnancies are more likely to be lost. (Personal interview, January 2013)

These considerations lead the gynecologist to the conclusion that it is necessary that an agency act as a specialized intermediary because in the do-it-yourself search by intentional parents for a surrogate mother, this important issue is not always taken into account. The lawyer, on her side, always mentions to her clients (both intended parents and surrogate mothers) this potential source of conflict:

> Every time I say: "Before you choose a surrogate, when you are interviewing them, ask them how they feel about reduction, termination. You have to make sure, ask a lot of questions about that." A lot of people don't consider Down syndrome in the contract, and most people wouldn't abort for that. We actually have to put that down in there. (Personal interview, January 2013)

The interviewee continues recounting a case of hers:

> I just had a surrogate who's doing… She's a niece of one of the parents, who are a gay couple, two men. And she's specifically said: "I would only carry one child, no matter what." Usually they carry at least two. And I said: "Even if it's identical twins?" They're both in the same amniotic sack [this occurs rarely, in less than 1% of natural conceptions]. And she said: "Look, they can hire a professional, I am doing it as a favor." She's not getting paid. And they had to accept.
> Every time you have at least twins, you have a higher risk, you might go on bed rest for the last month… She didn't want to put her body through that, basically. Usually you don't get people who would not carry twins, you might get people who would not carry triplets. (Personal interview, January 2013)

The contractual obligation is knowingly used in favor of the intended parents, as she quite candidly states:

> Everybody has been cleared by psychologists. And even medical clinics are requiring that. They have to make sure the parents and the surrogate don't have any diseases they are going to pass on to the child or to the surrogate. So, once cleared, they go to the lawyers, that means us, we draft the contract, which covers everything from the intention of the parties, making sure they understand law in California, making sure they understand law could change in California while they are pregnant, making sure they talked about and write down abortion, when they would abort, when they would not abort, when they would do a reduction for triplets, twins, and when they would not. It's not constitutional to enforce that, to make someone have an abortion or make them not have an abortion. But you can say: if you have an abortion, you have to pay them back or you can say... Usually you agree that if there are significant genetic defects, you agree to abort the child, and it's a parents' decision. And you usually say that if the parents and the doctor decide that, if you are carrying triplets, it's bad for your health, you reduce to two or one, based upon what the parents and doctor decide. The surrogate has to give those healthcare decisions about the baby to the parents. There's always something in there, tho', that says that if the surrogate is endangered, she makes the choice about aborting or about reducing from multiple to one, and also the financial ramifications for breaching that. You cannot enforce someone to physically to reduce or to abort the child, or not to. It's a constitutional right over your own body. But you try to make it sound like they have to. The contracts are getting longer and longer and there are lifestyle prohibitions, so they are trying to say you can't drink coffee, they don't want artificial sweeteners, so it grows and grows. (Personal interview, January 2013)

The gynecologist, too, when talking about "risk" means the situation unfavorable to the intended parents, as when we talked about the ethics of contracts:

> *Q: From my point of view, what is most controversial is the possible reaction of the surrogate mother, who after the pregnancy does not want to relinquish her parental rights. Have there been cases of this?*
> A: No, because we do... mostly we do gestational services, where the woman only gets the egg and the egg is not from her. And all the surrogates also have children of their own, you cannot be a surrogate and not have children. I mean, it's not a law but it's good medical practice, and it's the guidelines, so... And they're counseled extensively that it's not their child, and in California the Supreme Court made the decision that in this situation, the woman who carries the pregnancy is not the mother, so they do not have the legal right to keep the child. Now, traditional surrogacy is more risky because they provide the egg and the uterus and other states maybe do not have such a favorable legal climate as we have here, so people come from other states because there maybe their contracts are not enforceable, valid, you can challenge them. But in California it is not going to work, the legislation is so that you're going to lose it. (Personal interview, January 2013)

The surrogacy contract, in California and elsewhere, aims to give to intended parents disproportionate powers over the woman who is available to carry a pregnancy to term for them, even trying to appropriate her constitutional right to abortion. This is exactly what surrogate motherhood is like in Israel:

though surrogates are protected by the patients' rights law and cannot be forced to agree to such an intervention, refusal is considered a breach of the surrogacy contract. Surrogates are therefore implicitly forced to comply because they would otherwise have to reimburse a couple for all payments made until that point and to pay them an additional fine amounting to thousands of shekels.

The surrogate is also contractually obligated to take any medicine prescribed by the doctor exactly as instructed. Not taking a prescribed medication as indicated can constitute a breach of contract. On her part, if she wants to take any drug at all, even an aspirin, she must first ask the doctor's permission. If the fetus is in danger, the surrogate can be ordered hospitalized or confined to bed rest for any portion of the pregnancy. [...]

Even in the most amicable surrogate-couple relationship, tensions often arise over issues concerning the surrogate's body. [...] Couples routinely became upset if their surrogate wanted to travel by car or bus to a distant location while pregnant with their child. [...] surrogates also reported arguments with their couples over their conduct while pregnant, such as going out to pubs, taking their medicines at the appropriate times, and not answering their cell phones every time the intended mother called. (Teman 2010, 88–89)

The conclusion of Elly Teman is that:

These women are definitely subject to control of their bodies by state, legal, and medical institutions. Moreover, in a certain sense, they passively have things "done to" them by doctors (IVF, medicalized childbirth), by the state (which selects them to serve as instrumental womb replacements for infertile, married women), and by their couples, with whom they sign legal contracts that constrain their actions and may even harm their basic human right to govern their own bodies. (Teman 2010, 192)

The social result of the existence of these contracts (but paid agreements have the same effect), is the strengthening of a particular interpretation of the practice of surrogacy: the one that sees the biological mother as a belly at the disposal of "clients," often to be deleted from the family history after having been used as a container. She is a body who must obey orders, without expressing any will relative to its "content," as this is regarded as the property of others. She is a worker doing the work of a slave. This instrumental interpretation of surrogacy is the opposite of the altruistic motives with which many women volunteer to become surrogate mothers, something they could do without submitting themselves to the obligations of a contract.

But the technology of IVF is there: should we resign and admit that women have been reduced to the inhuman status of vessels for developing the babies appropriated by richer people? Or should we try to use the force of the state to repress it outlawing a possibility of gain for women who have no better way (in their own or in their family's eyes) to make a living? I think we should regulate the situation in order to guarantee the possibility of generosity, while avoiding the construction of markets in babies, and repressing the existing ones.

Conclusion: ethical surrogacy

> Patriarchy needs somehow to institute fatherhood as indisputable fact, and in complementary fashion to render motherhood a matter of ideas—about what children really need, about who mothers are, about which women can be considered "fit" mothers and which unfit, about the secret, raw and therefore antisocial interior of the sacred and profane bond between mother and child.
>
> Ann Oakley

> I argued that regardless of the differences among us, all women must care about social and legal constructions of motherhood. Although we may make individual choices not to become mothers, social construction and its legal ramifications operate independent of individual choice.
>
> Martha Fineman

> Paradoxically, the biological mother may be disappearing at the same time as the biological father is reaching his apogee.
>
> Yasmine Ergas

> However, de facto surrogacy remains as legal as ever. All a man has to do is convince a woman to marry him; all a couple have to do is convince a love-starved and self-destructive woman to be their surrogate uterus for *free*.
>
> Phyllis Chesler

> The bourgeois clap-trap about the family and education, about the hallowed co-relation of parents and child, becomes all the more disgusting, the more, by the action of Modern Industry, all the family ties among the proletarians are torn asunder, and their children transformed into simple articles of commerce and instruments of labour.[153]
>
> Marx and Engels

Coming to the conclusions, a review of our initial definition is necessary: before and after IVF with donor eggs the tune has changed about the whole

---

[153] Quotations from Oakley's introduction to Chesler 1988, xvii; Fineman 1995, 51; Ergas 2012a.; Chesler 1988, 158; Karl Marx and Friedrich Engels: *Manifesto of the Communist Party*, 1948 https://www.marxists.org/archive/marx/works/1848/communist-manifesto/ch02.htm accessed 5.2.2015.

question of genetic descent. The realization of the full potential of this technique has been slow: it did not appear immediately, or rather it was not immediately exploited in this way, but by now we have reached the point where genetic unrelatedness of a "contract child" (which has also been called a "designer child") has fully entered the social horizon of the wealthier part of humanity, a commodification also promoted by anti-discriminatory legal reasoning. I will now exclude this case, redefining the practice of surrogate motherhood as the agreement that a birth mother makes to relinquish her parental rights and let a baby *genetically related* to one or two intended parents be brought up in their family without her. This definition is more restrictive than the initial one, which also contemplated genetic unrelatedness. But in the course of our exploration we have discovered how close surrogacy is to adoption. In terms of relationships, they can be distinguished only by the genetic relatedness of the developing child. Birthing a baby totally unrelated to intended parents makes it undistinguishable from an adopted child, simultaneously unmasking the "intended parents" as adoptive parents. "Surrogacy" in these cases must be treated not just in analogy to adoption, but as a clear—and clearly unethical—case of it: it can't even fall under adoption regulations because it is forbidden (and wrong) to make an agreement to intentionally bring a child into the world just to be adopted, especially (but not only) if money changes pockets (see also Radin 1996). The prohibition of this kind of gestational surrogacy could be feasible, since labs and doctors must be involved to perform phoney surrogacy/real adoption of a child still to be conceived, and since in all countries it is unpalatable to risk losing a medical license for the pricey high-tech labs needed to perform IVF, it would also be effective.

We have seen that birth mothers in surrogacy entertain and act upon many different ideas of motherhood. On one side there are those who act according to the value of donating happiness to others, choosing to sacrifice themselves for a bigger purpose. They conceive of the baby as unrelated to them. On another side there are the workers, who accept or are forced into an agreement to gain money, hoping to be offered other advantages, such as the opportunity to migrate to a richer country. There are of course all the possible mixes of the two motivations in each woman. A few of these women then move to yet another position: the vision of a unity of mother and child that it is wrong and hurtful to separate: they decide to exit the agreement, or would like to. The progress in technology has been used to obfuscate that what is really happening in these gestations is what always has. "If the egg does not belong to the gestating woman, she is therefore unessential. She is not the mother, we need to redefine what a mother is," is the hocus-pocus to make the pregnant woman disappear. But she is there and she is not an incubator, she feels, thinks, and wants to decide. She is the birth mother, and she will take decisions that everybody else must pay respect to.

On the side of the intended parents there can be all kind of attitudes: I have no doubt that many "egalitarians" (as Ragoné calls them in contrast to the "pragmatists") respect the decisions of the surrogate mother, treating her well and maintaining respectful contact during pregnancy and after, as mothers generally value it. But especially in contracts the tendency to impose the intended parents' will is evident, perhaps implicit in the self-sacrificing role of the surrogate. Intended parents justify their pretensions with their disbursement of money. It is in order to save it or to enter into more favorable agreements that some rich, or middle-class people from rich countries go abroad, running the risk of creating "suspended babies" who will suffer even more if juries do not act in a humanitarian way, condoning their unlawful actions. Some intended parents claim that surrogacy is always ethical if one only avoids the countries where exploitation appears obvious. Others simply choose the cheaper option.

The subjective meaning of surrogacy for the woman and for these intended parents stretches apart as much as the social and economic gap between them. These visions are difficult to reconcile, especially if a contract makes intended parents feel entitled to a "product" in the form of the delivery of a (healthy) child. The contract encourages the intended parents to consider the birth mother as a worker. If it is valid, they are legally allowed to expropriate her of her "product," even if the subjective experience of the surrogate mother is not that she has been working for somebody else, but doing a good deed, giving the gift of life to people who can't have children of their own (but if other people are making money out of it, I would certainly consider her an exploited worker, despite her subjectivity[154]). She is in fact doing an exceptional act, that can be asked and hoped for but not re-

---

[154] I think we can safely agree that exploitation can happen also when the subject, the worker, does not perceive it. The problem of creating class consciousness derives exactly from these misperceptions.

quired, coming from exceptional women in exceptional circumstances. The approach of the intended parents should be the respect of the true will of the woman who goes through the pregnancy process—regardless of whom the ovum belonged to. This would also mean that, from the ethical point of view, surrogacy should not be considered work, that is, as an obligation. If women are forced to do it through economic necessity and would argue for a right to work in this way, there are two reasons to refuse it. The first is the protection of the rights of laborers, by not accepting the legalization of work that is invasive of the body to such a degree. The second reason—if the labor rights of women are already compromised, as in poor countries—is that this job amounts to baby-selling, with a detrimental effect on society.

But anything can become a product, even friendship, as Arlie Hochschild has shown in her work *Outsourcing the Self* (2013). In the contemporary US the marketization of personal relationships is so advanced that even "friendship" can be bought at Rent-a-Friend agencies. Why not babies? Because Arlie Hochschild has also shown how deeply unsettling the recourse to markets for creating intimate connections is. We strive for authenticity as the best way to live our lives, despite being surrounded by the lies of money, as in Karl Marx's depiction:

> I am bad, dishonest, unscrupulous, stupid; but money is honoured, and hence its possessor. Money is the supreme good, therefore its possessor is good. Money, besides, saves me the trouble of being dishonest: I am therefore presumed honest. I am *brainless,* but money is the *real brain* of all things and how then could its possessor be brainless? Besides, he can buy clever people for himself, and is he who has power over the clever not more clever than the clever? Do I not, who thanks to money am capable of *all* that the human heart longs for, possess all human capacities? Does my money not, therefore, transform all my incapacities into their contrary?[155]

But this is not authenticity. We strive for the truth and for what is right and we strive to feel natural emotions in the same way as we strive for mental and physical health. There are commodities—goods and services—that we accept because everybody else does, because they are pillars of contemporary capitalist society, such as cheap meat and private cars, but once we open our eyes to realise and care about how things are produced, if we see nature and workers exploited, we cannot close them anymore, we must change.

---

[155] Karl Marx, *Economic and Philosophic Manuscripts of 1844*, "The Power of Money" (https://www.marxists.org/archive/marx/works/1844/manuscripts/power.htm accessed 21.1.2015). After "has" I omitted a note: "[In the manuscript: 'is'.—*Ed.*]."

The money given to the surrogate creates a "contract child" even where contracts are not valid. Public policy cannot endorse the selling of babies, nor permit the psychological burden imposed on them as grown-ups. It is not easy to find out what "contract children" think. Despite what Zelizer said about the normalcy of mixing money and affection, to be a contract baby does not seem acceptable at least to some of the grown-ups who have had this origin—though the voices that have publicly expressed themselves are few and more research is surely needed. It is well known that "Baby M" terminated her birth mother's rights as an adult and that she declared to the press to be happy to have been raised by the Sterns. Nevertheless she did not express herself against her birth mother, nor did she explain the reasons to legally cut her off. What is clear is only that she did not want to become a public figure as an adult because of her vicissitudes as a baby. People who do want to talk about their "contract child" origin are few and not so positive about the process:

> It looks to me like I was bought and sold. You can dress it up with as many pretty words as you want. You can wrap it up in a silk freaking scarf. You can pretend these are not your children. You can say it is a gift or you donated your egg to the IM [intended mother]. But the fact is that someone has contracted you to make a child, give up your parental rights and hand over your flesh and blood child. I don't care if you think I am not your child, what about what I think! Maybe I know I am your child. When you exchange something for money it is called a commodity.[156]

This is clearly the view of a child of traditional surrogacy, but the same conclusion that commodification, rather than a service as a sort of baby-sitter during pregnancy applies, was expressed by a young woman in the documentary *Breeders* by Jennifer Lahl (2014): "I have been bought," concludes Jessica Kern. Her origin from a gestational surrogacy agreement with gametes from other people was kept hidden from her by her abusive family. When she found out, she added this injury to all the others she had suffered. Now she keeps a blog and she's a vowed anti-surrogacy activist.[157]

In another sad moment of *Breeders*, Heather relates how the then 5-year-old child she had carried for an infertile couple asked her why she did not keep her like her other children. She also recounts her own moment of consciousness about the injustice of her separation from the baby when her

---

[156] Quote from the blog "Son of a Surrogate" http://theothersideofsurrogacy.blogspot.it/ accessed 13.10.2014.
[157] *The Other Side of Surrogacy* http://theothersideofsurrogacy.blogspot.it/ accessed 13.1.2015.

eldest daughter questioned her choice, having grown attached to the new baby her mother was expecting. A Catholic website gives a good write-down of this story:

> Another surrogate said it was her daughter who opened her eyes to the oddity of the situation. Already a mother of two who had enjoyed both pregnancies and had easy births, the woman said she felt that offering the use of her womb to an infertile couple would be a compassionate thing to do, along with helping her to pay her bills and stay home with her kids. But she hadn't counted on the emotional attachment her eldest daughter would form with her unborn half-sibling.
> "She loved babies," the surrogate said. "I mean, what was I thinking? I had two daughters at that point, and when my second daughter was born, it was the biggest thing that had happened in her life. It was like the best thing in the whole world to her. How on Earth did I think I could just give one away, and that she would be okay with it?"
> That same surrogate—who has a relatively open relationship with the adoptive family—later recounted the experience of visiting her surrogate daughter for the first time at the couple's home, some two months after the birth. The baby had been colicky and sleepless, crying for hours a night from the moment she had been removed from her birth mom at five days old. Within minutes of being placed in the surrogate's arms, she was fast asleep on her chest, seemingly content for the first time in weeks.
> "At no point did I consider how it would affect her," the surrogate said, "being a baby, spending, you know, nine months in my womb, and then five days in my arms, and then being taken away."
> Five years later, on a visit to her birth mom's house, that little girl would look at her three half-siblings and observe that she looked more like her birth mother than any of them did.
> "She looked right at me, innocent as could be, and said, 'We have the same hair, and we have the same eyes,'" the surrogate recalled. "'Why did you give me away and keep them?'" (Andersen 2014)

Elizabeth Anderson sums up the question: "The unsold children of surrogate mothers are also harmed by commercial surrogacy. The children of some surrogate mothers have reported their fears that they may be sold like their half-brother or half-sister, and express a sense of loss at being deprived of a sibling" (Anderson 1990, 78). Like someone has said, paid surrogacy is like selling Joe to be able to send Susan to college.

Only private and free agreements guarantee the values of the practice: offering to gestate a baby as an act of generosity. The current policy of the Netherlands, with the birth mother's decision after birth and only documented pregnancy-specific expenses can be paid for by the intended parents, seems to be a good example. How can we express altruism, even self-sacrifice, in a way that is not an expression of oppression in a patriarchal context, but that really means that these values are important for us? This is a real theoretical and practical problem, and I think it can only be solved by leaving open the possibility of free surrogacy agreements. But the agreement must be private, that is, without third parties fostering it, and not enforceable by the state. And the cultural critique of women's position in these agreements must not cease. The distorted view of reality called "false consciousness" by Marxists and by second wave feminists does exist (George Annas in 1990 called surrogacy a "powerful deception"), and in steering society in one or the other direction cultural battles are of utmost importance. People do act contrary to at least some of their collective interests, as they belong to different groupings, choosing to primarily belong to one at the detriment of the others—and in the case of surrogate motherhood, false consciousness sees generosity towards new families in cases where women's capacities are exploited: women are persuaded, or persuade themselves, to carry out an emotionally and physically dangerous act just in order to feel appreciated. My cultural critique is that surrogates are not offering "to gestate a baby," but they offer the baby itself, mistakenly intending it as an act of generosity. Their agency must nevertheless be recognized, as a voluntary and gratuitous agreement cannot be prohibited on grounds of false consciousness, while the prohibition of surrogacy as a job should be. Law is the embodiment of social struggle, and the line delimiting prohibition of commercial contracts and paid agreements preserves women's labor rights, canceling surrogacy from the kinds of work that are acceptable. Feminists in India, where these labor rights are already lost, are divided between those who still fight against surrogacy, highlighting its unacceptable conditions, those who are advocating for harm-reduction policies that would lift the condition of surrogates, and those who think of surrogacy as a resource that should be freely used by women (Sarojini and Dharashree 2010). In Israel feminists are strongly against what happens there:

> We believe that surrogacy in Israel should be prohibited. At the least, surrogacy must not be allowed to become an accepted, routine procedure, and should provide a solution only in rare, very extreme cases. (Lipkin and Samama 2010, 3)

The social meaning of the legal configuration of surrogacy in Israel is dismal:

> Removing the social, bureaucratic and economic barriers from the application for surrogacy strengthens the message that motherhood should be the center of a woman's life.
> It makes the acceptance of one's infertility less and less legitimate and increases the social and family pressure on women and couples to invest all their resources in the attempt to achieve parenthood.

> The widespread accessibility to surrogacy harms the currently existing social perceptions of the importance of the relationship between the mother and the baby in her womb, and conveys a social message that this relationship has no actual emotional and legal significance. (Lipkin and Samama 2010, 5–6)

As in Israel—and even in countries without contracts—if we allow the altruist to pocket some money for their inconvenience we end up on a slippery slope: at the end of the day a market in babies has likewise sprung up. Undoubtedly, the battle against commercial surrogacy, "altruistic" contracts, and paid agreements is part of the battle against the commodification of everything, from health services to education, from communications to water and all the other services that in welfare states we used to call public. And to preserve the birth of children from its appropriation by market forces is not only a part of the anti-capitalist battle, but a position widely shared by all those who want to protect human dignity and defend the freedom of pregnant women.

The same values of choice and agency that must allow for a voluntary and gratuitous form of surrogacy agreements, decisively impede the admissibility of the contract, aimed at rescinding with the force of the state the mother/child relationship. This is what Paola Tabet and Christine Delphy worry about: that the recognition of the biological importance of the mother/child relationship would condemn women to serve their children as if parenthood were a pure biological fact and not a social arrangement, that currently requests reproductive work only from women even as a part of their gender identity. But I do not think that a bettering of the social position of women, and a fairer division of labor within heterosexual families can be accomplished by denying the importance of the archetypal Mother/Child dyad, symbolically based on care and dependency of the newborn on its natural source of nourishment. Parenthood is in no way a simple biological fact—but pregnancy is, and the supremacy of the birth mother in establishing families must be recognized, especially by feminists. The rights of fathers and mothers are often unjustly leveled by law, in a matter where the woman has a nurturing, creative, indivisible and also often difficult and painful "relationship" with the egg fused with sperm becoming a baby, while everybody else, including the genetic or the social father/mother, have only an indirect one. I envision an ethic that puts relationships in the first place, relationships that are based primarily on human choice, but also on natural ties—that can be chosen because they are recognized as coming from the body, which is not our enemy but ourselves.

In cross-border surrogacy laws we are witnessing a "race to the bottom" similar to that of outsourcing capitalist production. States with laws permitting the transfer of parental authority by contract undermine the capacity of other states to uphold the principle *mater semper certa est*. The European Court of Justice established in 2014 a worrying precedent affirming the validity of birth certificates that falsely declare motherhood, encouraging regulations of surrogacy. To counter this blow—the umpteenth neoliberal move by the EU—an international convention should be formulated within the framework of the UN—not by private entities like The Hague Conference, which wants to recognize the laws of the "lowest bidder" and accept every demeaning condition out of a well-crafted fear of imaginary stateless babies. Its direction must be the opposite: a ban on commercial surrogacy in line with the ban on commercial adoption, fighting not only *improper* but *all* gains (that is: *improper gains*), to stop marketing babies (a measure advisable in international adoption, too). The visas for surrogacy should be granted only with the guarantee that the country of origin accepts the agreements, and that crossing borders with a newborn and its foreign-issued birth certificate is legal.

Overall, we must be aware that it is contrary to commonsense, and certainly not in the interest of the child—as also established in international conventions recognizing the right to family life—to conceive a child in order to separate it from its mother. If a birth mother however decides for the separation (also in adoption conventions, family life is protected "as far as possible"), she can always do it with a private agreement. Genetic-only motherhood should be put on a par with fatherhood in the possibility of recognizing a child (if its mother consents), since with the advent of IVF a legal change is necessary to end the dispute about the mother's position by the two or three women involved (egg contributor, gestational mother, intended mother). Technology has made possible a distinction that should be recognized on birth certificates: born of a birth mother, with X and Y's genetic contribution (if they are not anonymous), with the parenting right pertaining at birth to the birth mother and her affiliates.

Surrogacy is a process that touches lives very intimately, and I am not contesting the depth of the feelings of people who want to reproduce, nor do I want to deny the genuine joy of couples that find their much desired sons and daughters through the help of women who gestate for them, but intended parents should really be the first to make sure they are not stealing somebody else's baby, as the woman having it is its mother. A failure to recognize this is unethical, just an exercise in class and money privileges.

That said, something is wrong in our culture about reproduction. Childless individuals or couples are interrogated about their motives, they must justify their choices, as having kids is deemed the normal—a word meaning "compulsory"—situation. This is one important reason why the infertile suffer. The positive concept of being childfree, free to pursue other goals in life other than just reproducing the social order (children are seldom nonconformists and, if they grow up sufficiently free, more often than not start to rebel against their parents in their teens), should become much more popular than it now is (Diehl 2014). Women should feel valued for their personal qualities and not just for their birthing capacities ("This was the one thing I was good at," recalls Kim Cotton in her book). And infertility is still seen as a woman's guilt: the patriarchal mind considers women useful insomuch as they bring forth their husband's male children, his replicas, into the world.[158]

But in this historical phase there is no general interest to multiply humans. We must get rid of the pro-natalist attitude that has been part of the religious teaching in most parts of the world with the intent of multiplying followers by the cultural transmission of religious tenets, deeply rooted as learned in childhood. The root of the problem is that—against any lucid evaluation of the situation of the human species on this planet—religions, cultures, tradition, social conformity, even the media and academia pundits are strongly pushing people to feel incomplete if they do not marry and start a family. Our society is pervaded with a rhetoric of the "happy ending" of forming a family. Marrying and having children is the ultimate certificate of normality: "After marriage, what else if not babies?" declared two Chicano gays in the news, shown happily playing with their twin daughters at home.

---

[158] In India status is generally still conferred to brides only when they deliver a male heir, necessary for religious reasons. Only after this "proof" of their womanly capacities are they integrated into the family, deserving the others' respect: "A woman is respected as a wife only if she is mother of a child, so that her husband's masculinity and sexual potency is proved and the lineage continues" (Government of India 2009, 6).

But we should stop blaming the "childless" and celebrate the "child-free," contributing to diminishing the unsustainable impact of the capitalist world-economy on Earth, and to reducing the workforce (as in the birth strikes—*la grève des ventres*—in the 20s). But especially in the core countries a nationalistic alarm is instead sounding about the diminution of the birth rate (happening all over the world, if the UN statistics are to be trusted). This really sounds ridiculous especially as core countries are depleting Nature's resources at a faster and faster pace. So the first prerequisite to a fairer stance towards ourselves and Nature would be to acknowledge that there is no social need for such a large number of kids as human beings altogether are still having, and to encourage people to have less of them, or leave reproduction out entirely, particularly if their bodies are not capable. Infertility is not an illness, and surrogacy is not a therapy. In a model other than the current privatization of affection by "the sexual family" with its isolated living arrangements, the childless could participate in parenthood—there is no surplus of care, that must instead be paid for. This is a fact in our money-driven economy, but a fact that children are unable to comprehend. Barbara Katz Rothman unmasks the fiction of "money substituting for relationships" in child care:

> Someone has to actually, truly, literally be there with them. Whoever that person is—mother, father, adoptive parent, sibling, housekeeper, teacher, baby-sitter, day-care worker, grandparent—whoever is with that child, that person must never be thought of as being there in place of someone else. The person who is there, is there. The person is not a substitute-someone-else. The person caring for a child is in a first-person, one-on-one, direct relationship to that child. That relationship deserves respect, just as that work deserves to be valued. And respect, as we know from what has happened to mothers historically, is not adequately taken care of with politeness and a Mother's Day card. It must come with legally recognized rights. Someone who has been raising a child has moral rights invested in that child. At a minimum, we have to protect child-care workers from arbitrary firing, from loss of visitation rights to the children they raise, from having the relationship with the child used as a source of exploitation. (Katz Rothman 1989, 103 and 2000, 144)

And that relationship starts in the womb. A new human life is formed by the fusion of two gametes, two "seeds," that mature inside a man's and a woman's body. But it is the woman that receives the male one, detached from him with sexual pleasure, and eventually also the female one, detached with surgery and pain. It is the female body that makes the conglomerate of cells grow into a newborn, generally with ache and suffering. It is her flesh and her blood that nurture the little creature from invisibility to the different stages of development, finally pushing the baby, mature after nine months of pregnancy, outside her uterus, through her vagina, out into the light and the air, finally capable of breathing and actively searching for her or his food—again mother's milk. Considering the relationship on the future baby's side, she is the only human being whom the new child knows profoundly.

Long gone are the times when women were worshipped for their birthing capacities (some say it never happened...), when the "language of the Goddess" expressed itself in symbols of the feminine, in the Paleolithic statuettes of motherly ripeness—huge breasts and buttocks—objects of wonder and adoration for the continuity of life and Nature. Women's procreative power has been harnessed to male needs, subjugated to masculine gods. Women have been enslaved in patriarchy, obliged to give birth to the male heir of their masters, on their conditions. We are struggling against all this, in order to regain power over our lives, in order to be able to make choices. We still endeavor to be seen as human on equal footing with males, the heirs to the patriarchal tradition that values them more than females—and women are still forced to bear those heirs. But today children are only necessary to the fetish of "economic growth," that is, the expansion of capital: they are the workforce and the consumers of the future, needed in growing numbers to perpetuate the ceaseless capitalist cycle that, unfearful of clashes, reduces everything to money, disregarding ecology and humanity—and especially *womanity*.

References

Achmad, Claire. 2013. "New Zealand." In *International Surrogacy Arrangements: Legal Regulation at the International Level*, edited by Katarina Trimmings and Paul Beaumont, 295–310. Oxford: Hart Publishing.

ACOG (The American Congress of Obstetricians and Gynecologists). 2005. "ACOG Committee Opinion 324: Perinatal Risks Associated with Assisted Reproductive Technology." *Obstetrics and Gynecology* 106:1143–1146 (reaffirmed 2007). http://www.acog.org/Resources-And-Publications/Committee-Opinions/Committee-on-Obstetric-Practice/Perinatal-Risks-Associated-With-Assisted-Reproductive-Technology

Alexander, Latashia S. 2006. *I'm Having Their Baby: a Guide to the Gestational Surrogate*. Instantpublisher.Com, USA.

Andersen, Kirsten. 2014. "Girl with a Korean Mom Thought She Was Adopted. The Truth Was More Unsettling." *LifeSite*, June 25. https://www.lifesitenews.com/news/child-of-surrogacy-speaking-out-against-so-called-donor-conception.

Anderson, Elizabeth S. 1990. "Is Women's Labor a Commodity?" *Philosophy and Public Affairs* 19:71–92.

Annas, George J. 1988. "At Law: Death Without Dignity for Commercial Surrogacy: The Case of Baby M." *The Hastings Center Report 18(2):* 21–24.

Annas, George J. 1990. "Fairy Tales Surrogate Mothers Tell." In *Surrogate Motherhood: Politics and Privacy*, edited by L. Gostin, 43–58. Bloomington: Indiana University Press.

Badiale, Marino, and Massimo Bontempelli. 2010. *Marx e la Decrescita. Perché La Decrescita Ha Bisogno del Pensiero di Marx*. Trieste: Abiblio.

Bakalar, Nicholas. 2011. "I.V.F. Brings a Slightly Higher Cancer Risk." *New York Times* 7 Nov. http://www.nytimes.com/2011/11/08/health/research/ivf-brings-slightly-higher-risk-for-ovarian-cancer.html?_r=0

Balcom, Karen A. 2011. *The Traffic in Babies: Cross-Border Adoption and Baby-Selling between the United States and Canada, 1930—1972*. Toronto: University of Toronto Press.

Baslington, Hazel. 2002. "The Social Organisation of Surrogacy: Relinquishing a Baby and the Role of Payment in the Psychological Detachment Process." *Journal of Health Psychology* 7(1): 57–71.

Bequaert Holmes, Helen. 1986. "Surrogacy with IVF Carries Biological Risks." *The Hastings Center Report* 16(4): 49.

Berend, ZsuZsa. 2010. "Surrogate Losses: Understandings of Pregnancy Loss and Assisted Reproduction among Surrogate Mothers." *Medical Anthropology Quarterly* 24(2): 240–262.

Bertschi, Nora. 2014. *Leihmutterschaft: Theorie, Praxis und rechtliche Perspektiven in der Schweiz, den USA und Indien*. Bern: Stämpfli.

Bhandar, Brenna. 2015. "Title By Registration: instituting property and conjuring racial value in the settler colony." *Journal of Law and Society. (In Press)*

Botti, Caterina. 2007. *Madri cattive : una riflessione su bioetica e gravidanza*. Milano: Il Saggiatore.

Brännström, M., Johannesson, L., Bokström, H., Kvarnström, N., Mölne, J., Dahm-Kähler, P., Enskog, A., Milenkovic, M., Ekberg, J., Diaz-Garcia, C., Gäbel, M., Hanafy, A., Hagberg, H., Olausson, M., Nilsson, L. 2014. "Livebirth after uterus transplantation." *The Lancet* 385. http://www.thelancet.com/journals/lancet/article/PIIS0140-6736%2814%2961728-1/ppt

Brazier, M., Campbell, A., Golombok, S. 1998. *Surrogacy: Review for Health Ministers of Current Arrangements for Payments and Regulation - Report of the review team*. Department of Health, London.

Bulletti, C., Palagiano, A., Pace, C., Cerni, A., Borini, A., De Ziegler, D. 2011. "The Artificial Womb." *Annals of the New York Academy of Sciences* 1221: 124–128.

Chesler, Phyllis. 1988. *Sacred Bond: The Legacy of Baby M*. New York: First Vintage Books.

Ciccarelli, Janice C., and Linda J. Beckman. 2005. "Navigating Rough Waters: An Overview of Psychological Aspects of Surrogacy." *Journal of Social Issues* 61(1): 21–43.

Corti, Ines. 2000. *La maternita per sostituzione*. Milano: Giuffrè.

Cotton, Kim, and Denise Winn. 1985. *Baby Cotton*. Milano: Frassinelli.

Crawshaw, Marylin, Blyth, Eric, and Van den Akker, Olga. 2013. "The Changing Profile of Surrogacy in The UK—Implications for National and International Policy and Practice." *Journal of Social Welfare and Family Law* 34(3): 265–275.

Dalla Costa, Mariarosa and Selma James. 1972. *The Power of Women & the Subversion of the Community*. Bristol: Falling Wall Press.

Danna, Daniela. 2009. *Stato di Famiglia : Le Donne Maltrattate di Fronte alle Istituzioni*. Roma: Ediesse, 2009.

Danna, Daniela. 2014. "Population Dynamics and World-Systems Analysis". *Journal of World Systems Research* 20(2): 207–228. http://www.jwsr.org/wp-content/uploads/2014/08/Danna_Vol20_no2.pdf

Diehl, Sarah. 2014. *Die Uhr, die nicht tickt: Kinderlos glücklich; eine Streitschrift*. Zürich: Arche, 2014.

Druzenko, Gennadiy. 2013. "Ukraine." In *International Surrogacy Arrangements: Legal Regulation at the International Level*, edited by Katarina Trimmings and Paul Beaumont, 357–366. Oxford: Hart Publishing.

De Araujo, N., Vargas, D., de Campos Velho Martel, L. 2013. "Brazil." In *International Surrogacy Arrangements: Legal Regulation at the International Level*, edited by Katarina Trimmings and Paul Beaumont, 85–92. Oxford: Hart Publishing.

Dillon, Nancy. 2012. "Noted Surrogacy Lawyer Theresa Erickson Sentenced for her Role in Baby-Selling Scheme." *NY Daily News*, February 24. Accessed December 28, 2014. http://www.nydailynews.com/news/crime/noted-surrogacy-lawyer-theresa-erickson-sentenced-role-baby-selling-scheme-article-1.1028320

Dunaway, Wilma A., ed. 2014. *Gendered Commodity Chains: Seeing Women's Work and Households in Global Production*. Stanford: Stanford University Press.

Dworkin, Andrea. 1983. *Right-Wing Women*. New York: Perigee Books.

Ekman, Kajsa E. 2013. *Being and Being Bought: Prostitution, Surrogacy and the Split Self*. Melbourne: Spinifex Press.

Ergas, Yasmine. 2012a. *The Transnationalization of Everyday Life: Cross-Border Reproductive Surrogacy, Human Rights and the Re-visioning of International Law.* (12 March 2012) Institute for the Study of Human Right: Columbia College. http://hrcolumbia.org

Ergas, Yasmine. 2013. "Thinking 'Through' Human Rights: The Need for a Human Rights Perspective With Respect to the Regulation of Cross-border Reproductive Surrogacy." In *International Surrogacy Arrangements: Legal Regulation at the International Level*, edited by Katarina Trimmings and Paul Beaumont, 427–436. Oxford: Hart Publishing.

Faraoni, Alicia B. 2002. *La Maternità Surrogata: la Natura del Fenomeno, gli Aspetti Giuridici, le Prospettive di Disciplina.* Milano: Giuffrè.

Federici, Silvia. 2012. *Revolution at Point Zero: Housework, Reproduction, and Feminist Struggle.* Oakland: PM Press.

Fernandes, Camila P. 2014. "Maternidade substituta - uma visão geral acerca da sua licitude frente ao Código Civil, ECA e Código Penal Brasileiro." *Conteudo Juridico, Brasilia-DF*: 24.6.2014. http://www.conteudojuridico.com.br/artigo,maternidade-substituta-uma-visao-geral-acerca-da-sua-licitude-frente-ao-codigo-civil-eca-e-codigo-penal-brasi,48755.html#_ftnref9

Field, Martha A. 1988. *Surrogated Motherhood.* Harvard: University of Harvard Press.

Fineman, Martha A. 1991. *The Illusion of Equality. The Rhetoric and Reality of Divorce Reform.* Chicago and London: The University of Chicago Press.

Fineman, Martha A. 1995. *The Neutered Mother, the Sexual Family and Other Twentieth Century Tragedies.* New York: Routledge.

Fineman, Martha A. 2009. "The Sexual Family." In *Feminist and queer legal theory: intimate encounters, uncomfortable conversations*, edited by Martha Albertson Fineman, Jack E. Jackson, Adam P. Romero, 45–64. Farnham ; Burlington: Ashgate.

Folbre, Nancy, and Julie A. Nelson. 2000. "For Love Money—or Both?" *The Journal of Economic Perspectives* 14(4): 123–140.

Folbre, Nancy. 2001. *The Invisible Heart: Economics and Family Values.* New York: The New Press.

Folbre, Nancy. 2009. *Greed, Lust and Gender: A History of Economic Ideas.* Oxford: Oxford University Press.

Frediani, Jodi. 1982. "A Short History of Childbirth." In *The Birth Book.* Tree Press. (Second edition)

Gamble, Natalie. 2012. "Should Surrogate Mothers Still Have an Absolute Right to Change their Minds?" *BioNews* 678. http://www.bionews.org.uk/page_196180.asp

Garrity, Amy. 2000. "A Comparative Analysis of Surrogacy Law in the United States and Great Britain - A Proposed Model Statute for Louisiana." *Louisiana Law Review* 60: 809–830.

Golombok, Susan E. and Clare E. Murray. 2003. "Families created through surrogacy: Parent-child relationships in the first year of life." *Fertility and Sterility* 80(3):50.

Ghosh, Aditya. 2006. "Cradle of the World". *The Hindustan Times*, December 24. http://www.hindustantimes.com/news-feed/nm21/cradle-of-the-world/article1-195533.aspx

Gilbert, Scott F. 2014. "A Holobiont Birth Narrative: The Epigenetic Transmission Of The Human Microbiome." *Frontiers in Genetics.* 19 August.

Golombok, S., Blake, L., Casey, P., Roman, G., Jadva, V. 2013. "Children Born through Reproductive Donation: A Longitudinal Study of Child Adjustment." *Journal of Child Psychology and Psychiatry* 54: 653–660.

Golombok, S., Casey, P., Readings, J., Blake, L., Marks, A. & Jadva, V. 2011. "Families created through surrogacy: Mother-child relationships and children's psychological adjustment at age 7." *Developmental Psychology.* 47(6):1579–1578.

Golombok, S., Murray, C., Jadva, V., MacCallum, F.& Lycett, E. 2004. "Families Created Through Surrogacy Arrangements: Parent-Child Relationships In The First Year Of Life." *Developmental Psychology.* 40:400–411.

Golombok, S., Murray, C., Jadva, V., Lycett, E., MacCallum, F. & Rust, J. 2006. "Non-genetic and non-gestational parenthood: Consequences for parent-child relationships and the psychological well-being of mothers, fathers and children at age 3." *Human Reproduction.* 21:1918–1924.

Goslinga-Roy, Gillian. 2000. "Body Boundaries, Fiction of the Female Self: An Ethnographic Perspective on Power, Feminisim, and the Reproductive Technologies." *Feminist Studies* 26(1): 113–140.

Göttner-Abendroth, Heide. 1980. *Die Gottin und ihr Heros. Die matriarchalen Religionen in Mythos, Märchen und Dichtung.* München: Frauenoffensive.

Govan, Fiona. 2006. "Ban on Surrogacy Creates Trade in 'Wombs for Rent'." *The Telegraph*, August 1. http://www.telegraph.co.uk/news/1525347/Ban-on-surrogacy-creates-trade-in-wombs-for-rent.html.

Graff, Nicole B. 2000. "Intercountry Adoption and the Convention of the Right of the Child: Can the Free Market in Children be controlled?" *Syracuse Journal of International Law and Commerce* 27(2): 405–430.

Hatzis, Aristides N. 2009. "From Soft to Hard Paternalism and back: the Regulation of Surrogate Motherhood in Greece." *Portuguese Economic Journal* 8: 207.

Hatzis, Aristides N. 2010. "The Regulation of Surrogate Motherhood in Greece" http://www.google.it/url?sa=t&rct=j&q=&esrc=s&source=web&cd=1&ved=0CC4QFjAA&url=http%3A%2F%2Fwww.researchgate.net%2Fprofile%2FAristides_Hatzis%2Fpublication%2F228145584_The_Regulation_of_Surrogate_Motherhood_in_Greece%2Flinks%2F02bfe50eb0d66216ef000000.pdf&ei=MbieVOTYPMiBU6T3gaAL&usg=AFQjCNFeDjNYkPHuFxlwD7b0-kq81WiTJg&bvm=bv.82001339,d.d24&cad=rja retrieved 27.12.2014.

Hibino, Yuri, and Yosuke Shimazono. 2013. "Becoming a Surrogate Online: 'Message Board' Surrogacy in Thailand." *Asian Bioethics Review* 5(1): 56–72.

Hochschild, Arlie R. 2012. *The Outsourced Self. Intimate Life in Market Times.* New York: Metropolitan Books.

Horsey, Kirsty. 2010. "Challenging Presumptions: Legal Parenthood and Surrogacy Arrangements." *Child and Family Law Quarterly* 22(4): 449–474.

Huo, Zhengxin. 2013. "The People's Republic of China." In *International Surrogacy Arrangements: Legal Regulation at the International Level*, edited by Katarina Trimmings and Paul Beaumont, 93–104. Oxford: Hart Publishing.

Inhorn, Marcia C. 2010. "'Assisted' Reproduction in Global Dubai: Reproductive Tourists and Their Helpers." In *Globalized Motherhood*, edited by Wendy Chavkin and JaneMaree Maher, 180–202. New York: Routledge Press.

Ingram, John D. 1993. "Surrogate Gestator: A New and Honorable Profession." *Marquette Law Review* 76: 675–684.

Jadva, V., Casey, P., Blake, L. & Golombok, S. 2012. "Surrogacy families ten years on: Relationship with the surrogate, decisions over disclosure and children's understanding of their surrogacy origins." *Human Reproduction*. 27:3008–3014.

Jadva, V., Murray, C., Lycett, E., MacCallum, F. & Golombok, S. 2003. "Surrogacy: The experiences of surrogate mothers. *Human Reproduction*. 18 (10):2196–2204.

Kane, Elizabeth. 1989. "Surrogate Parenting: A Division Of Families, Not A Creation." *Reproductive and Genetic Engineering: Journal of International Feminist Analysis* 2(2) http://www.finrrage.org/pdf_files/RepTech%20General/Surrogate_Parenting_Kane.pdf

Keyes, Mary. 2013. "Australia." In *International Surrogacy Arrangements: Legal Regulation at the International Level*, edited by Katarina Trimmings and Paul Beaumont, 25–48. Oxford: Hart Publishing.

Khazova, Olga. 2013. "Russia." In *International Surrogacy Arrangements: Legal Regulation at the International Level*, edited by Katarina Trimmings and Paul Beaumont, 311–324. Oxford: Hart Publishing.

Johnson, Suzanne M., and Elizabeth O'Connor. 2002. *The Gay Baby Boom: the Psychology of Gay Parenthood*, 97. New York: New York University Press.

Katz Rothman, Barbara. 1989. "Women as Fathers: Motherhood and Child Care Under a Modified Patriarchy." *Gender and Society* 3(1): 89–104.

Katz Rothman, Barbara. 2000. *Recreating Motherhood: Ideology And Technology In A Patriarchal Society.* New York: Norton

Katz Rothman, Barbara. 2012. "Book review: Teman, E. Birthing a Mother." *Sociology of Health & Illness* 34(3):475–480.

Krimmel, Herbert T. 1992. "Can Surrogate Parenting be Stopped? An Inspection of the Constitutional and Pragmatic Aspects of Outlawing Surrogate Mother Arrangements." *Valparaiso University Law Review* 27:1–38. http://scholar.valpo.edu/vulr/vol27/iss1/1

Lamm, Eleonora. 2013a. "Mexico." In *International Surrogacy Arrangements: Legal Regulation at the International Level*, edited by Katarina Trimmings and Paul Beaumont, 255–272. Oxford: Hart Publishing.

Landes, William M., and Richard A. Posner. 1978. "The Economics of the Baby Shortage." *The Journal of Legal Studies* 7(2): 323–348.

Lipkin, Nuphar, and Etti Samama. 2010. *Surrogacy in Israel. Status Report 2010 and Proposals for Legislative Amendment.* Isha L'Isha - Haifa Feminist Center. http://isha.org.il/wp-content/uploads/2014/08/surrogacy_Eng001.pdf

London, Catherine. 2012. "Advancing a Surrogate-Focused Model of Gestational Surrogacy Contracts." *Cardozo Journal of Law & Gender* 18: 391–422.

Lothian, Judith A. 2000. "Why Natural Childbirth?" *Journal of Perinatal Education* 9(4): 44–46.

Lynn Budin, Stephanie. 2011. *Images of Woman and Child from the Bronze Age: Reconsidering Fertility, Maternity, and Gender in the Ancient World.* Cambridge: Cambridge University Press.

MacCallum, F., Lycett, E., Murray, C., Jadva, V. & Golombok, S. 2003 "Surrogacy: The experience of commissioning couples. *Human Reproduction.* 18 (6):1334–1342.

Imrie, S., Jadva, V. & Golombok, S. 2012. "The long-term psychological health of surrogate mothers and their families." *Fertility and Sterility.* S46, 98.

Makuch, Maria. 2010. "Maternal positions and mobility during first stage of labour." *RHL Commentary. The WHO Reproductive Health Library.* Geneva: World Health Organization. http://apps.who.int/rhl/pregnancy_child birth/childbirth/routine_care/CD003934_makuchmy_com/en/index.html

Markens, Susan. 2007. *Surrogate motherhood and the politics of reproduction.* Berkeley: University of California Press

McDermott, Hannah. 2012. "Surrogacy Policy in The United States and Germany: Comparing the Historical, Economic and Social Context of Two Opposing Policies". *Senior Capstone Projects* 137. http://digitalwindow.vassar.edu/cgi/viewcontent.cgi?article=1137&context=senior_capstone

McIntosh, Tania. 2012. *A Social History of Maternity and Childbirth: Key Themes in Maternity Care.* London: Routledge.

Meyer, Catherine. 2005. *Le Livre noir de la psychanalyse. Vivre, penser et aller mieux sans Freud.* Paris: Les Arènes.

Oakley, Ann. 1986. *The Captured Womb: A History of the Medical Care of Pregnant Women.* New York: Basil Blackwell (Original edition 1984).

O'Donohoe, S., Hogg, M., MacLaran, P., Martens, L., Stevens, L. 2014. *Motherhoods, Markets and Consumption: The Making of Mothers in Contemporary Western Cultures.* New York: Routledge.

Ohs, Alayna. 2002. "The Power of Pregnancy: Examining Constitutional Rights in a Gestational Surrogacy Contract." *Hastings Constitutional Law Quarterly* 29: 339–372.

Oliver, Kelly. 1989. "Marxism and Surrogacy." *Hypatia* 4(3): 95–115.

Pande, Amrita. 2010. "'At Least I Am Not Sleeping with Anyone': Resisting the Stigma of Commercial Surrogacy in India." *Feminist Studies* 36(2): 292–312.

Pande, Amrita. 2014. *Wombs in Labor. Transnational Commercial Surrogacy in India.* New York: Columbia University Press.

Parker, Philip. 1982. "*Surrogate Motherhood*: The Interaction of Litigation, Legislation and Psychiatry." *International Journal of Law and Psychiatry* 5: 341–354.

Parker, Philip. 1983. "Motivation of Surrogate Mothers: Initial Findings." *American Journal of Psychiatry* 140: 117–18.

Pauknerová, Monika. 2013. "Czech Republic." In *International Surrogacy Arrangements: Legal Regulation at the International Level*, edited by Katarina Trimmings and Paul Beaumont, 105–118. Oxford: Hart Publishing.

Perreau-Saussine, Louis, and Sauvage, Nicolas. 2013. "France." In *International Surrogacy Arrangements: Legal Regulation at the International Level*, edited by Katarina Trimmings and Paul Beaumont, 119–130. Oxford: Hart Publishing.

Peterson, Iver. 1987. "Surrogate Mothers Vent Feelings of Doubt and Joy." *The New York Times,* March 2. http://www.nytimes.com/1987/03/02/nyregion/surrogate-mothers-vent-feelings-of-doubt-and-joy.html

Phillips, Anne. 2013. *Our Bodies, Whose Property?* Princeton: Princeton University Press.

Pimentel, David. 2001. "Biomass utilization, limits of." In Vol. 2 of *Encyclopedia of Physical Science and Technology* : 159–171. San Diego: Academic Press.

Place, Jeffrey M. 1994. "Gestational Surrogacy and the Meaning of 'Mother': Johnson v. Calvert, 8511 P.2d 776 (Cal. 1993)" *Harvard Journal of Law & Public Policy* 17(3): 907–918.

Posner, Richard A. 1987. "The Regulation of the Market In Adoptions." *Boston University Law Review* 67: 59–72.

Posner, Richard A. 1989. "The Ethics of Enforcing Contracts of Surrogate Motherhood." *Journal of Contemporary Health Law and Policy* 5: 21–31.

Rae, Scott B. 1994. *The Ethics of Commercial Surrogate Motherhood: Brave New Families?* Westport: Praeger.

Ragoné, Helena. 1994. *Surrogate Motherhood: Conception in the Heart.* Boulder: Westview Press.

Ragoné, Helena. 1996. "Chasing the Blood Tie: Surrogate Mothers, Adoptive Mothers and Fathers." *American Ethnologist* 23(2): 352–365.

Raymond, Janice G. 1990. "Reproductive Gifts and Gift Giving: The Altruistic Woman." *The Hastings Center Report* 20(6): 7–11 http://www.questia.com/library/1G1-9267490/reproductive-gifts-and-gift-giving-the-altruistic

Raymond, Janice G. 1994. *Women As Wombs: Reproductive Technologies And The Battle Over Women's Freedom.* North Melbourne: Spinifex.

Regalia, Anita, Colombo, Grazia, Pizzini, Franca. 1984. *Mettere Al Mondo : La Produzione Sociale Dei Parto.* Milano: F. Angeli.

Rethimiotaki, Eleni. 2008. "A comparative gendered reading of changes in kinship law after the regulation of reproductive technology," In *Gender, Body and the Gendered Difference: the Encounter of Law and Social Theory*, edited by Marina Maropoulou, 49–65. Athens: Athens University and European Program of Gender and Equality Studies.

Rethimiotaki, Eleni. 2015. "'Commercialization trends and the legal nature of the female body: 'unholy' comparisons of prostitution with surrogating mothering in postmodern Greece." Paper presented at the conference *Troubling Prostitution*, Vienna, 16–18 April 2015.

Rivkin-Fish, Michele. 2013. "Conceptualizing Feminist Strategies for Russian Reproductive Politics: Abortion, Surrogate Motherhood, and Family Support after Socialism. ' *Signs* 38(3): 569–593.

Robertson, John A. 1983a. "Procreative Liberty and the Control of Conception, Pregnancy, and Childbirth." *Virginia Law Review* 69(3): 405–464.

Robertson, John A. 1983b. "Surrogate Mothers: Not So Novel After All". *Hastings Center Report* 13: 28–34.

Robertson, John A. 1986. "Embryos, Families, and Procreative Liberty: The Legal Structure of the New Reproduction." *South California Law Review* 59: 939–948.

Rokas, Konstantinos A. 2013. "Greece." In *International Surrogacy Arrangements: Legal Regulation at the International Level*, edited by Katarina Trimmings and Paul Beaumont, 143–166. Oxford: Hart Publishing.

Sama (Resource Group for Women and Health). 2012. *Birthing A Market: A Study on Commercial Surrogacy.* New Delhi.

Sanger, Carol. 2007. "Developing Markets in Baby-Making: In the Matter of Baby M." *Harvard Journal of Law and Gender* 30: 67–97.

Sarojini, N.B., and Dharashree Das. 2010. "ARTs: Voices from progressive movements." In *Making babies : birth markets and assisted reproductive technologies in India,* edited by S. Srinivasan, 22–43. New Delhi: Zubaan Books.

Scuola di Barbiana. 1967. *Lettera a una Professoressa.* Firenze: Libreria Editrice Fiorentina.

Shakargy, Sharon. 2013. "Israel." In *International Surrogacy Arrangements: Legal Regulation at the International Level,* edited by Katarina Trimmings and Paul Beaumont, 231–246. Oxford: Hart Publishing.

Shanley, Mary L. 1993. "'Surrogate Mothering' and Women's Freedom: A Critique of Contracts for Human Reproduction." *Signs* 18(3): 618–639.

Sherman, Ted. 2011. "N.J. Gay Couple Fight for Custody of Twin 5-year-old girls." *The Star-Ledger* http://www.nj.com/news/index.ssf/2011/12/nj_gay_couple_fight_for_custod.html

Shultz, Marjorie M. 1990. "Reproductive Technology and Intent-Based Parenthood: an Opportunity for Gender Neutrality." *Wisconsin Law Review* 297.

Slabbert, Melodie and Christa Roodt. 2013. "South Africa." In *International Surrogacy Arrangements: Legal Regulation at the International Level,* edited by Katarina Trimmings and Paul Beaumont, 325–345. Oxford: Hart Publishing.

Smerdon, Usha R. 2008. "Crossing Bodies, Crossing Borders: International surrogacy between the United States and India." *Cumberland Law Review* 39: 15–85.

Smerdon, Usha R. 2013. "India." In *International Surrogacy Arrangements: Legal Regulation at the International Level,* edited by Katarina Trimmings and Paul Beaumont,187–218 . Oxford: Hart Publishing.

Smietana, Marcin. 2013. "Las paternidades y maternidades en las familias de padres gays creadas por gestación subrogada," In *Maternidades, Procreación Y Crianza En Transformación* , edited by Carmen López, Diana Marre, Joan Bestard, 203–220. Barcelona: Edicions Bellaterra.

Snyder, Steven H. 2013. "United States of America." In *International Surrogacy Arrangements: Legal Regulation at the International Level*, edited by Katarina Trimmings and Paul Beaumont, 387–396. Oxford: Hart Publishing.

Spandrio, Roberta, Regalia Anita and Giovanna Bestetti. 2014. *Fisiologia Della Nascita : Dai Prodromi Al Post Partum*. Roma: Carocci Faber.

Spitz, Elie. 1996. "'Through Her I Too Shall Bear a Child': Birth Surrogates in Jewish Law." *The Journal of Religious Ethics* 24: 65–97.

Sullivan, E.A., Zegers-Hochschild F., Mansour R., Ishihara O., de Mouzon J., Nygren K.G., Adamson G.D. 2013. "International Committee for Monitoring Assisted Reproductive Technology (ICMART) World Report: Assisted Reproductive Technology 2004." *Human Reproduction* 28(5):1375–90. http://www.icmartivf.org/icmart-world-report-art-2004.pdf

Tabet, Paola. 1998. *La Construction Sociale de l'Inégalité des Sexes. Des Outils et des Corps*. Paris: L'Harmattan.

Tabet, Paola. 2014. *Le dita tagliate*. Roma: Ediesse.

Teman, Elly. 2010. *Birthing a Mother: The Surrogate Body and the Pregnant Self*. Berkeley: University of California Press.

Thompson, Chris. 2013. "And Baby Makes Four." *California Lawyer,* January: 14–21.

Tieu, Matthew M. 2009. "Altruistic Surrogacy: the Necessary Objectification of Surrogate Mothers." *Journal of Medical Ethics* 35: 171–175.

Trimmings, Katarina, and Paul Beaumont. 2013. "General Report on Surrogacy." In *International Surrogacy Arrangements: Legal Regulation at the International Level*, 439–550. Oxford: Hart Publishing.

Utian, W.H., et al. 1985. "Successful Pregnancy After an In-vitro Fertilization-embryo Transfer from an Infertile Woman to a Surrogate." *The New England Journal of Medicine* 313: 1351.

Van den Akker, Olga. 2007. "Psychosocial Aspects of Surrogate Motherhood." *Human Reproduction Update* 13(1): 53–62.

Van Leeuwen, F.E., et al. 2011. "Risk of borderline and invasive ovarian tumours after ovarian stimulation for in vitro fertilization in a large Dutch cohort." *Human Reproduction* 26(12): 3456–3465.

Van Wesenbeeck, Ine. 1994. *Prostitutes' Well Being and Risk*. Amsterdam: VU University Press.

Vora, Kalindi. 2010. "Medicine, Markets and the Pregnant Body: Indian Commercial Surrogacy and Reproductive Labor in a Transnational Frame." *Scholar and Feminist Online* 9 http://sfonline.barnard.edu/repro tech/vora_01.htm

Vora, Kalindi. 2009. "Indian Transnational Surrogacy and the Commodification of Vital Energy." *Subjectivities* 28(1): 266–278.

Vora, Kalindi. 2013. "Potential, Risk, and Return in Transnational Indian Gestational Surrogacy." *Current Anthropology* 54.

Wallerstein, Immanuel. 2004. *World-Systems Analysis: An Introduction*. Durham: Duke University Press.

Weathers, Helen. 2008. "Now I Realise How Hopelessly Naive I Was to Become Britain's First Surrogate Mother, Admits Kim Cotton." *Daily Mail*, February.

Weis. 2014. 'Не страшно ничего, работа есть работа. [Not horrible at all, work is work]'. *Working as a 'Surrogate Mother' in Saint Petersburg. Seminar. Centre for Independent Social Research*. Saint Petersburg, Russia. September 2014.

Yamamoto, Kevin, and Shelby A.D. Moore. 2001. "A Trust Analysis Of a Gestational Carrier's Right To Abortion." *Fordham Law Review* 70: 94–186.

Zelizer, Vivian. 1985. *Pricing the Priceless Child*. New York: Basic Books.

Zermatten, Jean. 2010. "The Best Interests of the Child Principle: Literal Analysis and Function." *International Journal of Children Rights* 18(4): 483–499.

Zipper, Juliette, and Selma Sevenhuijsen. 1987. "Surrogacy: Feminist Notions of Motherhood Reconsidered." In *Reproductive Technologies : Gender, Motherhood And Medicine*, edited by Michelle Stanworth, 118–138. Cambridge: Polity Press, 1988.

***ibidem*-**Verlag

Melchiorstr. 15

D-70439 Stuttgart

info@ibidem-verlag.de

www.ibidem-verlag.de
www.ibidem.eu
www.edition-noema.de
www.autorenbetreuung.de